PROFESSIONAL COMMUNICATIONS IN EYE CARE

PROFESSIONAL COMMUNICATIONS IN EYE CARE

Ellen Richter Ettinger, O.D., M.S., F.A.A.O.
Associate Professor, Department of Clinical Sciences
State University of New York, State College of Optometry
New York

Foreword by

Mack Lipkin, Jr., M.D.
President and Chairman, American Academy
on Physician and Patient, Baltimore;
Associate Professor of Clinical Medicine and Director,
Division of Primary Care and Internal Medicine,
New York University Medical Center

Butterworth-Heinemann
Boston   London   Oxford   Singapore   Sydney   Toronto   Wellington

Library of Congress Cataloging-in-Publication Data

Ettinger, Ellen Richter.
   Professional communications in eye care / Ellen
Richter Ettinger.
      p. cm.
   Includes index.
   ISBN 0-7506-9306-1 (acid-free paper)
   1. Optometry—Practice. 2. Communication in medicine.
   I. Title.
RE959.E88   1993
617.7'5--dc20   93-6134
                                          CIP

British Library Cataloguing-in-Publication Data

A catalogue record for this book is available from the British
Library

Butterworth-Heinemann
80 Montvale Avenue
Stoneham, MA 02180

10 9 8 7 6 5 4 3 2 1

Printed in the United States of America

Dedicated to my husband, Dr. Henry Ettinger,
and my parents,
Harriet Richter and the late Louis Richter,
for their love, support, and never-ending inspiration.

Contents

Foreword

Professional Communications in Eye Care is the first empirically based communications text written for optometrists and provides an invaluable service for the optometry community. It may prove to be the most important book students study as optometrists-in-training.

Why are communication skills so important for the optometrist? Communication holds a prominent place in the work life: It is of central importance to the practice and is critical in patient care.

Depending on work rate and type of practice, a typical optometrist might expect to have 250,000 patient encounters in a forty-year career. This is an extraordinary number of times to do anything. It makes sense to try to maximize the effectiveness, efficiency, and satisfaction to be found in each of these encounters. Central to this goal is the effective use of communications skills.

Consider the importance of the medical interview to your practice. It has been shown repeatedly that the doctor–patient interaction is a major determinant of the doctor's satisfaction with the encounter, and by extension, with the practice. In other words, how you communicate will directly and substantially affect how happy you are in your work as an optometrist! Similarly, the doctor–patient interaction directly affects how satisfied the patient is with the encounter and with the doctor. Good communicators have satisfied patients—patients who both return for future visits and recommend the doctor to others. Because practices are built most often by word of mouth, the lesson is: *Good communications build successful practices.*

The interview is the central tool in patient care. It determines the accuracy and completeness of clinical data obtained from the patient and provides essential information about the patient both as a person and as a patient with a range of medical problems—many of which have critical importance in eye care. The interview also provides the optometrist with an understanding of how the patient may act as a partner in care: How the patient will cope with problems and comply with diagnostic and therapeutic interventions. In short, the interview is integral to almost every aspect of patient care.

Dr. Ettinger addresses the importance of building skills to maximize the value of the medical interview in *Professional Communications in Eye Care*. This novel approach for optometry combines an extensive knowledge of the empirical literature about the doctor–patient relationship, communications science, and the medical interview. This book is organized in a sensible progression of topics and features case studies chosen from eye care, including fear of blindness, fear of aging, cancer, and breaking bad news to patients.

Medical communications studies is a relatively new field that began in the modern era with the onset of easily available recording equipment, especially video recording. The first pioneering efforts were made by Barbara Korsch who videotaped over 800 interviews in an emergency room. Korsch's work demonstrated that communication frequently occurred in disparate languages and that patients and providers rarely understood each other. Since then, thousands of studies have extended and expanded on the work she started.

In the late 1970s, an organization called the Task Force on the Medical Interview and Related Skills became the "invisible college" for those in the medical communications world. The Task Force developed many services to the field including courses for teachers, collaborative research, a computerized bibliography, and a textbook entitled *The Medical Interview* (not yet published). In 1992, this Task Force became the American Academy on Physician and Patient. Dr. Ettinger then undertook massive individual study and preparation that have given the book both roots in the mainstream of Academy thinking and conceptualizing and her own creative additions.

Mastering the doctor–patient interview and relationship is a lifelong task one never completes. Begin it by developing a solid approach and good habits—this is the responsibility of each student and each introductory course. Acquire experience and continue to develop skills. Regularly monitor your work and correct bad habits and behaviors as needed. Audiotape or videotape yourself and review the tapes periodically to check communications skills.

It may be valuable to obtain another perspective: Enlist the help of a peer, mentor, or staff member to evaluate your skills or periodically attend a course in which skills are worked on in small groups where peer and expert feedback is readily available. Expand your knowledge of the field and the new concepts and findings by keeping up with current literature.

This lifelong process begins now with this book. *Professional Communications in Eye Care* is an excellent guide, for both the beginning student of optometry and the practicing optometrist, to use to facilitate thinking about and perfecting communications skills. May it serve you well in this most critical endeavor in your development as a doctor of optometry!

Mack Lipkin, Jr., M.D.

Preface

I first became aware of the impact of communications on medical care through a personal incident. I share this to demonstrate a learning experience I had, painful as it was, which hit home about the effects of a doctor's communication.

When I was in my third year of optometry school, my father had a stroke and was hospitalized. It was a mild stroke, and he was being monitored, but while he was in the hospital, he suffered another stroke. This one was a major stroke, and he was on and off a respirator for about a month. It was a very difficult and painful experience because I loved and adored my father.

One day, I observed that my father was having trouble breathing, and I asked the head resident to check on him. "Can you please check on my father?" I asked. "I think he is having some discomfort." The doctor barely looked up from his paperwork, and said that he would, but he appeared very busy and I wasn't confident that he would take the time to see my father.

After about an hour or so, when the doctor still had not checked on my father, I asked him again, very politely, if he would please check on my father. This time, he looked up from his paperwork, obviously upset at being interrupted, and said in a stern voice, "I can't waste my time with Mr. Richter. I have to spend my time with patients who can be helped." I will never forget the harshness of that message. His response transmitted two pieces of information to me: (1) he did not feel that my father was important or worth his time, and (2) my father was not going to make it. The weight of both statements was overwhelming, but the intensity of the second was the most severe. What a shocking way to find out that a loved one is not going to survive.

The thought of that resident's words still sends waves of shock through my body. He was obviously not skilled in communications and clearly had no idea of the effect of communications on the patient and the patient's family. I wish I could convey to him the long-lasting effect that his statement has had on me. If I could talk to him now, I would want to tell him that although health professionals must set priorities in attending to their patients, they do not have the right to judge the value of an individual.

In our own experiences as health care professionals, fortunately, not everyone will have to experience the impact of communications in the vivid, dramatic way that I did. It is my hope that my experience and *Professional Communications in Eye Care* illustrate the impact communications can have on patients, their families, and their care.

Do we ever appear less than supportive to a low vision patient who is mourning over her loss?

Do we ever sound less than compassionate to a parent who wants to understand why his child is not performing well in school?

Do we ever forget to attend to the fears of the patient newly diagnosed with glaucoma or cataracts?

Sometimes it is easy to get so caught up in staying on schedule and so used to patients' problems, that we forget to respond to their real experiences. We ask about pain, redness, and blurred vision. But do we ever ask about patients' fears, anxieties, or concerns?

I dedicate this book to one tired, overburdened resident who, in his own harsh way, taught me the importance of communications. I hope he has learned, and that others may too, that patients can be treated with love and compassion. This book was written with the hope that through improved communications, we can learn to provide better care to patients.

Acknowledgments

I would like to express my deepest gratitude and appreciation to Ms. Barbara Murphy, Ms. Karen Oberheim, and Ms. Kathleen Higgins of Butterworth-Heinemann. Their dedication and expertise have contributed significantly to this project. I also would like to express my appreciation to Ms. Claudia Perry and Ms. Irene Vito of the Harold Kohn Vision Science Library of the State University of New York (SUNY) State College of Optometry for their tireless efforts in obtaining references related to the topics in this text. My thanks also to Mr. Wayne Grofik and Ms. Diane Schiumo for their assistance.

This book is dedicated to my loving husband, Henry, and my wonderful family for their love, joy, and support. They make life so beautiful. Henry, you have always been a source of encouragement, strength, and support. And to my parents, who taught me to love, and to reach out to others, I thank you for giving me the gift of warmth.

How to Use
This Book

Part I of this book forms the base of the communication skills that doctors use in the health care setting. Models of communication (Chapter 1) and interviewing strategies (Chapter 2) introduce and lay the groundwork for these skills. Chapters 3 to 11, on topics including listening skills, nonverbal communication skills, building patient compliance, educating patients, interdisciplinary communications, and doctor–staff communications, build on the model and develop the skills needed to communicate in the clinical setting.

Part II applies communication strategies to specific patient groups. These groups, such as the non-English-speaking patient, the visually or hearing-impaired individual, the patient who abuses drugs or alcohol, and the victim of child or domestic abuse, present special communications challenges. The "nervous" patient, the "silent" patient, the "rambling" patient, and the "grief" patient all have clinical needs that must be met. One of the most fulfilling experiences for a clinician is helping a patient whom others may not have been able to reach. In these challenging situations, it is sometimes hard to know where to start. To help provide direction, strategies for interaction and case studies are presented.

Clinical cases throughout this book help to provide examples of good patient care. Although many textbooks use the form of Patient A.W. or Patient R.S., it was felt that a case with initials does not evoke the image of a real person. The use of proper names for patients reminds us that we deal daily with patients, not just cases. The names used, however, are not those of actual patients. Dale Carnegie once said that "a person's name is to that person the sweetest . . . sound." Using a patient's name is a way of demonstrating respect, and of showing that you recognize his or her identity. By giving the patients real names, with realistic needs and concerns, it is hoped that the cases attain optimal instructive value.

Introduction: Bridging the Art and Science of Clinical Care

Clinical care is a combination of two contributing forces: art and science. When closely interwoven, the two forces are strongest; either element alone is not as powerful as the two together. Knowing how to effectively combine the two aspects in the clinical setting is key to optimal patient care.

Developing a knowledge base and learning to manipulate clinical instruments is part of the science learned in school. Using the information gained through science to make meaningful contributions to the patient's life is an art learned through experience. Communication bridges art and science. Scientific results can be theoretically accurate but ineffective if they cannot be communicated to the patient. As technology and science become increasingly more complex, the doctor may find that focusing on the patient's perception of illness and disease takes more effort. Discovering how to explain complex technical information to the patient in a meaningful and appropriate way becomes more challenging. For each patient, the doctor must take what he or she knows from science and make relevant applications to the patient's life.

Part of the art of good clinical care is the development of a therapeutic relationship between the doctor and the patient. This doctor–patient rapport is a basic component of effective clinical intervention. To be able to discuss their symptoms and concerns, patients must first trust the doctor. Reading textbooks and articles cannot replace this facet of a doctor's care.

Students learn about disease and illness in the classroom and laboratory, but they can master patient care only by working and interacting with patients. *Professional Communications in Eye Care* attempts to bridge the gap between science and art by providing strategies to improve communication between the doctor and the patient. In this book, case studies are featured to illustrate actual communication strategies that can improve doctor–patient rapport.

The following recommendations can help the doctor interact with patients optimally:

1. Develop a sincere and genuine interest in each patient.
2. Use empathic listening and responding skills.
3. Greet the patient by name, and use the patient's name frequently throughout the clinical examination. Addressing a patient by name shows respect and a way of saying "I know you."
4. Communicate along both "factual" (cognitive) and "feeling" (affective) dimensions.
5. Listen with your eyes as well as your ears; communicate with your heart as well as your voice.
6. Use therapeutic touch when appropriate.
7. Learn to deliver bad news with sensitivity and compassion.
8. Understand a patient's pain and discomfort—recognize the patient's frustration when current science cannot provide an answer or a cure for the problem.
9. Never, never make a statement to the patient as fact unless you absolutely believe it to be true. Patients understand that doctors express opinions, but they should be labeled as opinion.
10. Remember that each patient is an individual with a unique set of needs. The doctor who can identify the individual concerns and goals of each patient will be most effective in addressing the patient's unique requirements.

Feinstein (1964) said that "to advance art and science in clinical examination, the equipment a clinician most needs to improve is himself." We can reach for the ophthalmoscope, the retinoscope, the slit lamp, and the tonometer, but to help the patient, we must first reach within ourselves. The following chapters address how the clinician can develop skills and abilities to interact optimally with patients. At the root of all good clinical care is the clinician who can use communication to bridge art and science.

REFERENCE

Feinstein AR. Scientific methodology in clinical medicine: IV. Acquisition of clinical data. Annals of Internal Medicine 61:1162, 1964.

Part I

Communication Skills

Models of Effective Communication

Good communication is the basis of effective doctor–patient interactions. Communicating well can make the patient more comfortable and confident in the doctor. Research has shown that patients who are more satisfied with their doctors are more likely to follow recommendations (Ley 1988). Poor communication can result in poor cooperation, participation, and compliance. In addition to demonstrating good clinical skills, the effective clinician must develop good doctor–patient communications.

Throughout the case history, testing sequence, and discussion of the diagnosis and management plans, the doctor must be able to share information and listen carefully to the patient. It is difficult for a patient to judge a doctor's competence in performing clinical tests, since most patients are not familiar with the precise methods and steps involved in clinical procedures such as ophthalmoscopy and tonometry. They are aware, however, when the interaction between the doctor and patient is not one that makes them feel comfortable and confident in the clinical environment. Achieving a positive doctor–patient rapport requires effective communications.

Communication is both an art and a science. The clinician who can master both aspects of communication can become more effective in gaining a patient's trust and cooperation.

MODELS OF COMMUNICATION

Several models of communication have been described (Gamble and Gamble 1987; Anderson 1990; Clampitt 1991; Schramm 1954; Shannon and

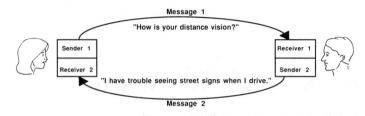

Figure 1.1 Model of communications. The cycle of communication involves a "sender" and "receiver" who transmit and receive messages.

Weaver 1949). Communication can be thought of as a cycle that involves a "sender" (speaker), a "receiver" (listener), and a "message" (a group of words that has meaning). For communication to be successful, all three components must be effective (Figure 1.1).

Clinicians who want to become better communicators should ask themselves three questions:

How can I become a better "sender"?
How can I become a better "receiver"?
How can I send "messages" that are clearer and more effective?

EXPANDING THE COMMUNICATIONS MODEL

The basic model of communication involving "sender," "receiver," and "messages" will be expanded to include context, channels, feedback, and noise, to provide a more complete account of the process of communication (Figure 1.2).

The Context

The context refers to the environment, or setting, in which communication takes place. Environments can affect the way we behave and communicate. Consider, for example, an examination room with loud, distracting noises in the background. The doctor and patient may have trouble hearing each other, and this will impact on the quality of the communication. Consider, as another example, an examination room that is very cold. Patients may feel very uncomfortable within that setting and may concentrate more on leaving the room than on what they are supposed to be doing while in the room.

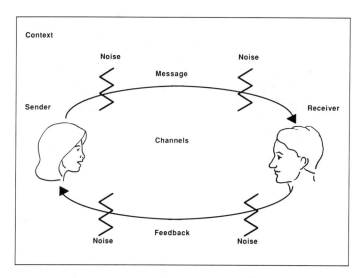

Figure 1.2 Components of communications. Communications involve the message, feedback, noise, channels, and context.

To increase the success of the doctor–patient encounter, the doctor should make an effort to make the patient comfortable and at ease, both physically and psychologically, so that the patient can concentrate on answering the doctor's questions and working with the doctor during the testing sequence. Making a patient comfortable is part of building good doctor–patient rapport, and is part of the "art" of good clinical care.

Channels of Communication

Communication can occur across the multiple channels of sound, sight, touch, smell, and taste. Awareness of multiple channels is a reminder that communication is not just limited to the words spoken by the doctor and patient. Eye contact, use of touch, and other nonverbal cues also affect the clinical interaction.

Feedback

Feedback refers to the verbal and nonverbal cues that are perceived in response to our communications. Feedback is a mechanism that can help identify obstacles to understanding between the doctor and patient.

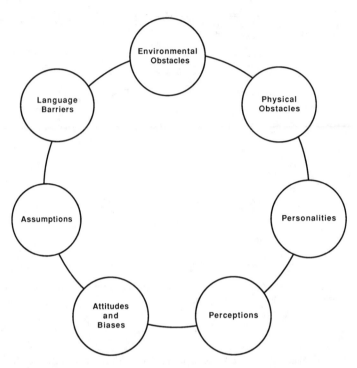

Figure 1.3 "The Wheel of Obstacles." The "Wheel of Obstacles" constantly turns and interferes with the flow of good communication. By eliminating obstacles and creating positive conditions for good communications, the doctor can optimize conditions for the doctor–patient interaction.

Noise

Noise can be described as anything that interferes with, impedes, or distorts a person's ability to send or receive messages. Potential sources of noise in the clinical environment can be demonstrated by the "Wheel of Obstacles" (Figure 1.3).

Noise in the clinical setting includes environmental obstacles (e.g., extreme cold or heat, loud background noises, poor lighting, uncomfortable office furniture), physical obstacles (e.g., hunger, pain), personality barriers, attitudes and biases, the patient's assumptions about the doctor, the doctor's assumptions about the patient, and other obstacles (e.g., language barriers). Anything that creates a barrier or obstacle to good communication is considered noise.

By being aware of the potential barriers in the clinical environment and eliminating these obstacles as much as possible, the doctor can create positive conditions for the doctor–patient interaction.

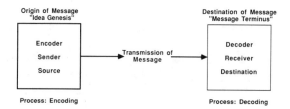

Figure 1.4 The encoder/decoder model. This model specifies the location of the message (origin or destination), the source (sender or receiver), and the process (encoding or decoding).

ENCODER/DECODER MODEL

The process of communication can also be described as a process of "encoding" and "decoding." The sender, the person who is transmitting the message, is the encoder; this person chooses words (encodes) to express the message. The receiver, who is the decoder, interprets the message (decodes) based on an understanding of the words that are spoken (Figure 1.4).

Sometimes miscommunication results when what the receiver decodes is not what the sender meant to encode. An example of this is when doctors are not conscious of the differences that can exist between their intended meaning and a patient's interpretation.

How can the message received by the listener be different from the speaker's intended message? When one person delivers a message to another person, the message can have several different forms (Gamble and Gamble 1987). Five different forms of a message are demonstrated in Figure 1.5. At each point in the communication process, the meaning of the message can be distorted, and information can be added or subtracted. The fourth message, the one that has been processed and analyzed by the listener, has a strong impact on the listener's interpretation. It is affected by the listener's attitudes, beliefs, and biases. The fifth message is the message that the listener will ultimately remember from the communication. Over time, this may change as a person's perceptions, perspectives, and impressions change. In the clinical environment, the fifth message will ultimately affect whether a patient remembers to follow up on a recommendation over time, and whether the patient remembers to perform the recommendation as prescribed.

Both the speaker and the listener can consciously, or unconsciously, modify the meaning as they encode and decode their messages. Sometimes we wonder why a listener does not understand what we say. We may not always be saying precisely what we are thinking, and the transmission does not always correspond directly with the intended message. Becoming

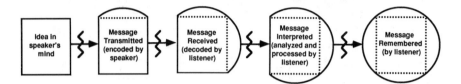

Figure 1.5 Potential changes in the meaning of the message. The message received by the listener does not always match the message intended by the speaker. Each arrow indicates a point at which a potential change in the meaning of the message can occur, where information can be added, deleted, or distorted. This illustration shows that the initial message intended by the speaker, represented by the square, gets changed along each step of the process, resulting in a final message represented by the circle. Both the speaker and listener can consciously and unconsciously modify information as they encode and decode their messages.

aware of potential gaps in encoding and decoding can make the sender more aware of the need to send clear, unambiguous messages.

APPLICATIONS OF MODELS OF COMMUNICATION IN THE CLINICAL SETTING

One method of looking at communications models applied in the clinical setting is to consider how the doctor functions as a "sender" and "receiver" in the clinical environment.

The Doctor as "Sender"

The doctor functions as a "sender" in many parts of the examination. During the case history session, the doctor must ask clear, understandable questions so the patient will know how to respond. If the patient does not understand what the doctor is asking, then the response from the patient will probably not meet the doctor's needs.

Throughout the examination, the doctor gives the patient instructional sets. These, too, must be clear for the patient to provide useful information. If the doctor wants a patient to focus on a distant target during retinoscopy, but the patient is actually looking at a near target, the clinical results may not be applicable to the doctor's intended use. Typical instructions for lateral phorias are "I'm going to show you two letters, one on the top and one on the bottom; tell me when they line straight up and down." If patients do not understand the directions, they may not know how to respond.

Providing additional explanations helps clarify instructional sets. "Tell me when the two letters line straight up and down, just like two buttons on a shirt." The description of two vertically aligned buttons gives the patient a visual context with which to understand the directions.

In cases in which verbal explanations are not understood, physical demonstrations may work. Demonstrations are particularly helpful when examining young children. For example, doctors may use their hands to represent the two letters, showing them separated both vertically and horizontally. Then, they move their hand to show how the two letters should line up, straight up and down, by physically holding one hand directly above the other. Some clinicians draw a picture showing what the letters look like before, and what they should look like when the results for the test are reached. Directions that are explained, described, or demonstrated effectively can improve the quality of the clinical information that is collected.

How to Become a Better "Sender"

- Orient communications to the needs of the patient (the "receiver").
- Ask clear, concise questions during the case history.
- Provide simple instructional sets.
- Use pictures or demonstrations to clarify instructions or directions.
- Provide understandable explanations of technical terms.
- Use language appropriate to the patient's understanding.
- Tailor speed of transmission to the patient's ability to process information.
- Use patient feedback to determine when further explanations and clarifications are necessary.
- Make sure nonverbal cues correspond to verbal communications.

Know Your Audience

When delivering a diagnosis to a patient, the doctor should explain the diagnosis clearly and accurately. "Knowing your audience" and subsequently orienting information to the patient's needs are primary rules of communications. A doctor may explain the same concept differently to different patients, depending on their background, knowledge, and experience. Knowledge of the patient's needs can help the doctor select the right words to describe a condition or disease process. As in discussing the diagnosis, presenting management plans optimally is largely a function of knowing the patient and knowing what motivates the patient to comply.

Use Language Appropriately

Throughout the examination, the doctor should use language that is appropriate to the patient's level of understanding. The most helpful cues in identifying the proper language to use with a patient are usually found by monitoring the patient's use of vocabulary and taking into account the patient's age and educational level. The doctor should avoid making stereotyped judgments and unfounded conclusions based on these data, however. By the time the doctor is ready to discuss the diagnosis and management plans with the patient, much information will already be available to provide insights into how best to communicate with the patient.

As in the use of language, speed of transmission is also a factor of "knowing your audience." People process information at different speeds. Obtaining a sense of how fast or slow you need to present information for a listener to comprehend you will increase the effectiveness of your message. Patient education is an area in which it is particularly important to tailor the message to the specific needs of the patient (see Chapter 8). Effective communicators know how to "read" their audience, so they can create effective messages.

Use Feedback to Guide Discussions with Patients

Feedback is probably one of the most underutilized elements of communication in clinical care. Using feedback is a crucial step that can provide the doctor with cues that further explanations and clarifications are necessary. As doctors and clinical students, we often consider that our primary responsibility is to give directions and recommendations to patients. Clinicians sometimes overlook valuable opportunities to identify areas of confusion and signs of poor compliance. By not taking the time to evaluate the patient's understanding and reactions, the clinician loses an opportunity to become a better communicator. By taking advantage of the full opportunities of feedback, the clinician can improve the outcomes of the clinical encounter.

The Doctor as "Receiver"

We often think of the doctor's function largely as one of giving information to patients—transmitting diagnoses, giving recommendations, and answering questions. Unless the doctor is also a good "receiver," however, the functions of diagnosing and designing appropriate management plans may be severely compromised.

By listening carefully to a patient's case history, the doctor will know how to ask appropriate follow-up questions that aid in differential diagnosis. Using feedback, the doctor can identify potential obstacles to compliance.

The doctor should also monitor the patient's nonverbal communications carefully. Nonverbal communications (e.g., eye contact, facial expressions, touch, gestures) and paralanguage (e.g., vocal intonation, speed of speaking, pitch, volume) are key components of the message. Although many people think of the message as the words that are used to transmit meaning, the accompanying nonverbal cues are also used to interpret what is said.

Miscommunication often results when nonverbal communications do not match verbal communications. For example, a doctor may tell a patient that something is "important," but the accompanying nonchalant, careless, or indifferent facial expressions or gestures suggest that what the doctor is saying is really not a priority. Being aware of verbal–nonverbal communication mismatches can also help the doctor identify patients who do not completely understand information that has been presented, or patients who are not fully committed to adhering to the doctor's recommendations. Examples include the patient who says "I understand, doctor," but who looks confused, or the patient who says "I clean my contact lenses almost every night," but the accompanying tone of voice and facial expression suggest that the level of compliance may be questionable. Nonverbal communications and paralanguage will be covered in detail in Chapter 4.

How to Become a Better "Receiver"

- Be an active listener.
- Attend to and project positive nonverbal communications.
- Eliminate distractions that impede effective communications.

Appear Interested in What the Patient Is Saying

The doctor who looks interested in what the patient is saying often appears more receptive to the patient. Many elements of nonverbal communications are involved and can demonstrate to the patient that the doctor is listening. For example, by maintaining eye contact with the patient during communication, nodding one's head, and demonstrating other receptive behaviors, the doctor can show interest in the patient's message. These factors will be covered in detail in the chapter on nonverbal communications (see Chapter 4).

Understand the Importance of Nonverbal Cues

By attending to the patient's nonverbal signs during the examination, the doctor can pick up important cues to communication.

A 76-year-old male presents for an eye examination. He is very quiet during the case history, avoiding much eye contact with the doctor. The doctor notices that he is tapping his foot on the floor anxiously. His facial expression is serious, and she observes that he is perspiring. Detecting that the patient is nervous, the doctor takes extra effort to put him at ease and asks if there is anything she can do to make the patient more comfortable.

Patients who are nervous, anxious, and apprehensive often demonstrate these feelings nonverbally. An astute doctor can improve the situation and build a therapeutic relationship with the patient.

Eliminate Distractions that Impede Effective Communications

Maintaining an interest in what the patient is saying can help keep your mind from wandering and from attending to other matters that are extraneous to the topic at hand. Preventing frequent phone calls and other interruptions is essential. Eliminating environmental barriers that can impede the communications process, such as loud background noises, can reduce the occurrence of distractions. Taking steps to eliminate these possibilities increases the probability of effective, productive communications.

How To Send Better "Messages"

- Be clear and concise.
- Explain technical terms.
- Orient the message to the audience.

Sending Effective Communications

The message is a set of words, but how can the message be improved? A good message should be clear and concise. Simplicity is the key to effective messages. Do not use complicated terms to impress patients; misunderstanding can result and patients may not understand what is wrong with them. When technical terms are used, they should be explained to make sure patients understand the diagnosis, and what follow-up actions are needed. Misunderstanding can cause a range of reactions from the opposite ends of the spectrum: panic (overreaction) and neglect (underreaction). In addition, misunderstanding can result in unnecessary fear and anxiety. By speaking in terms the patient can understand, the doctor can improve the messages that are sent, and ultimately the results that these messages produce.

The message should be complete enough to convey what is meant, but not so packed as to be "overloaded." Presenting the patient with a quantity of information that cannot be handled can result in confusion, dissatisfaction, and noncompliance.

In addition, the message should be geared to the audience. In clinical care, the "you-viewpoint" or "you-attitude" (Ceccio and Ceccio 1982) refers to the orientation of communications to the individual patient. The doctor's use of language and speed of transmission should reflect an understanding of the patient's needs.

Language and Communication

Language is an understood system, composed of words and symbols used to transmit meaning. The words or symbols within the message convey the meaning. Language is sometimes ambiguous, because words can often have different meanings to different people. If, for example, the doctor and patient use the same words to convey different meaning, then there will be misunderstanding and confusion between the two individuals.

The doctor has to be aware that patients may have preexisting beliefs and attitudes about certain clinical conditions and problems. For example, consider the term "cataract." What is a patient's reaction when you mention the word "cataract?" Many older people know other people who have had cataract surgery and thus may associate cataracts with surgery. Patients often assume that the diagnosis of cataracts means that they need to have surgery right away, if they are not explicitly told that this is not necessary.

Six-Step Communications Process

Communication can be described by two components: the process and the people involved. Sending messages can be considered a six-step process, from the generation of an idea or concept that a sender wants to communicate to the interpretation that the receiver makes of the message (Figure 1.6). The idea the speaker would like to transmit ("idea genesis") is "encoded" by identifying the words that will be used to convey the message. The message is transmitted by speaking to the receiver. The message is received as the sound waves reach the ears. Based on their experiences and understanding of the words, the receiver decodes and interprets the message.

The reverse direction of this process (feedback sent from the receiver to the sender in response to the message) can also be illustrated by this model (Figure 1.6). The first step in providing feedback to the sender is for the receiver to "respond to the message" that has been received. (This is an internal interpretation by the receiver.) The receiver may then "demonstrate signs" of response to the message. Nonverbal cues, such as a smile, a grin, or a look of confusion or doubt, may reflect the receiver's understanding or interpretation of the message. By learning to recognize and understand these signs, a speaker can become more attuned to whether a receiver understands the intended meaning of a message. The sender can

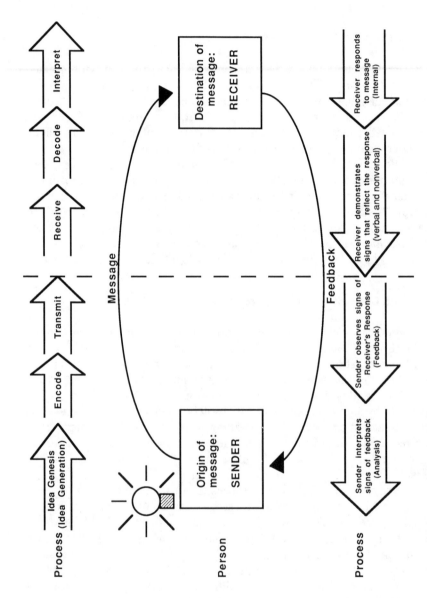

Figure 1.6 Six-step process and the feedback pathway. Communications can be illustrated as a process involving a group of steps.

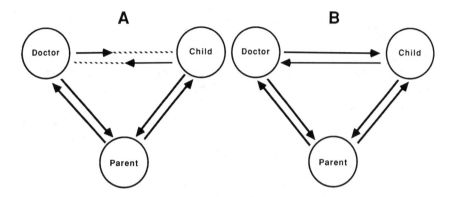

Figure 1.7 Three-way communications. When a parent brings a child in for an examination, three people are involved in the interaction: the doctor (D), the parent (P), and the child (C). The doctor should be conscious of the balance of communications across relationships. In A, the lines of communication are well balanced. In B, the doctor is directing most of the communication toward the parent. This can make the child feel alienated and apprehensive.

"observe the signs of the reader's response" and "interpret" them. Once this feedback loop is completed, the sender can send a new message to clarify, correct, or strengthen the intended meaning.

Who Is Communicating, and to Whom?

The basic communications model demonstrates one person as the sender and one as the receiver. The traditional examination in which the doctor is working with one patient is characteristic of this type of interaction. There are many cases, however, when several people are involved in a clinical encounter. Consider the following:

> A parent brings a 4-year-old child for an eye examination. There are now three people in the examination room: the parent, the child, and the doctor. The dynamics of the three-way exchange will have an impact on the effectiveness of the process. There are three possible communications relationships in this setting: communication between the doctor and the child, the doctor and the parent, and the parent and the child (Figure 1.7). Use of language, speed of transmission, and approach should vary for each relationship. Monitoring the balance of communications among these relationships, and the quality of the communication within each interaction, can make the doctor more sensitive to effective communications.

If all of the case history questions are directed to the parent, with the doctor rarely making eye contact with the child, the child may feel like a "nonperson" and fear or apprehension may result. The doctor has not given the child any sign that his or her feelings are important. The child becomes merely the "generator" of clinical data, and all emotional, "feeling" communication is carried out with the parent.

The doctor should be sensitive in maintaining an appropriate balance of communication with both the child and the parent. The appropriate balance is affected by the age of the child, the relationship between the parent and the child, and the relationship between the doctor and each individual. Working with children will be further elaborated in a chapter on communicating with pediatric patients (see Chapter 16).

> A 92-year-old patient presents for an eye examination. He is accompanied by his daughter, who observes the examination. The patient has a history of medical problems; both the patient and his daughter respond to case history questions.

As in the previous example, there are three possible communications relationships in this type of situation: the doctor and the patient, and doctor and the relative, and the patient and the relative. The balance and quality of communications should be monitored for all three relationships. When elderly patients come to the doctor with family members or caretakers, the qualities of the interaction with both the patient and relative are important. Ignoring the elderly patient, and addressing the case history and management plans to the caretaker, can make the patient feel like a child or a nonperson. A special section on working with geriatric patients is provided in Chapter 13 (pp. 184–187).

> A 57-year-old female who speaks a foreign language presents to the doctor's office with an interpreter. As typical in this type of clinical encounter, the doctor addresses most of the case history questions to the interpreter, who interacts verbally with both the patient and the doctor.

As in Figure 1.7, arrows can be drawn to illustrate the dynamics of the relationship among the three individuals: the interaction between the doctor and the patient, the doctor and the interpreter, and the patient and the interpreter.

The interpreter can be extremely helpful in conveying the needs of the patient. However, care must also be taken to maintain adequate eye contact and attention with the patient. In many cases, doctors ignore the patient almost entirely and attend to the interpreter for most of the examination. Failure to attend to the patient who speaks a foreign language can make the patient feel like a nonperson or a child. A discussion on communicating with patients who speak a foreign language appears in Chapter 13 (pp. 176–178).

When multiple family members and caretakers attend a clinical examination, the doctor has to remember to build a warm and therapeutic relationship with each of the individuals. Family support is often a key factor in gaining long-term cooperation and compliance.

STRATEGIES FOR IMPROVING COMMUNICATION IN THE CLINICAL ENVIRONMENT

It has been said that "you cannot not communicate" (Gamble and Gamble 1987). "Even if we . . . maintain absolute silence and attempt not to [communicate], our lack of response is itself a response;" therefore, it transmits meaning, "has message value, and hence communicates."

By knowing the components of good communication, clinicians can improve their ability to help patients. Good communication with the patient is the core of good clinical care.

1. Become a better "sender" and "receiver" in the clinical environment.
2. "Know the audience." By becoming more familiar with the patient, the clinician can have greater insights into which words should be used to (a) ask questions during the case history, (b) provide instructional sets for clinical procedures, (c) explain a diagnosis, and (d) present management plans. Cues in orienting communication to the audience include language used by the patient, age and educational level, the patient's speed of transmission, attitudes, and beliefs.
3. Be aware of a patient's nonverbal communications and paralanguage. These can often be subtle, but they are very helpful in identifying a patient's level of understanding.
4. Remember to watch for feedback. Becoming attuned to feedback from the patient can make the doctor much more effective in recognizing potential areas of confusion and in identifying possible obstacles to compliance.
5. Become more aware of the quality of communications in the clinical environment by watching clinical examinations, and evaluating the effectiveness of the interactions. A sample form for clinical observations is provided (Appendix A).

QUESTIONS FOR THOUGHT

1. How do you serve as a "sender" and "receiver" of information in the clinical environment? What other individuals are present in your environment (e.g., office staff), and how do they serve as communicators? If

you are a student, how do clinical faculty members serve as "senders" and "receivers" of information with you and patients?

2.   Other than listening to what patients say in words, how else can you learn about how they are responding to the clinical encounter? Other than in words, how do patients express when they are nervous? tired? uncooperative? uncomfortable?

3.   What are potential sources of "noise" in your clinical environment? How can you reduce or eliminate any effects that these sources may have?

4.   As described in this chapter, communications occur across multiple channels. Messages can be sent through sound, sight, touch, smell, and taste. During an interpersonal conversation with a friend or colleague, try to be aware of all of the messages that are sent across all channels. Do you think your consciousness across multiple channels increased the information that you gathered during this conversation? What information do you feel you would have missed if you attended only to the words of the speaker?

5.   Play a 10-minute part of a videotape (e.g., movie, television show) that includes an interpersonal conversation between two people. How do the individuals serve as "senders" and "receivers" of information? What channels are used to transmit information? Aside from using words, how do the individuals communicate?

6.   The characteristics of effective messages have been discussed in this chapter. Using these criteria to send effective messages, how would you explain the following terms to the patients listed?
   a.   Age-related macular degeneration (ARMD) to a 59-year-old female whom you have just diagnosed with ARMD.
   b.   Convergence insufficiency to a 34-year-old graduate student.
   c.   Dry eye syndrome to a 64-year-old woman who complains that her eyes tear.
   d.   Amblyopia to the parent of a 4-year-old child.
   e.   Posterior vitreous detachment to a 62-year-old patient who complains of a recent increase in floaters.
   f.   Keratoconus to a 19-year-old female whom you have just diagnosed as keratoconic.
   g.   Retinal hole to a 44-year-old patient with no symptoms.
   h.   Glaucoma to a 53-year-old patient with no symptoms.
   i.   Cataracts to a 67-year-old patient with blurred vision.

REFERENCES

Anderson CA. Patient Teaching and Communicating in an Information Age. Albany, NY: Delmar Publishers, 1990.

Ceccio JF, Ceccio CM. Effective Communication in Nursing Theory and Practice. New York: John Wiley, 1982.

Clampitt PG. Communicating for Managerial Effectiveness. Newbury Park, CA: Sage Publications, 1991.

Gamble TK, Gamble MW. Communication Works, 2nd ed. New York: McGraw-Hill, 1987.

Ley P. Communicating with Patients: Improving Communication, Satisfaction and Compliance. London: Croom Helm, 1988.

Schramm WL. How communication works. In Schramm W, ed., The Process and Effects of Mass Communication. Urbana: University of Illinois Press, 1954: 3–26.

Shannon C, Weaver W. A Mathematical Theory of Communication. Urbana: University of Illinois Press, 1949.

ADDITIONAL READINGS

DeVito JA. Human Communication: The Basic Course. New York: Harper & Row, 1988.

DeVito JA. Messages: Building Interpersonal Communication Skills. New York: Harper & Row, 1990.

Goodman GG, Esterly G. The Talk Book: The Intimate Science of Communicating in Close Relationships. New York: Ballantine Books, 1988.

Lipkin M, Putnam SM, Lazare A. The Medical Interview. New York: Springer-Verlag, 1993.

Tannen D. That's Not What I Meant! New York: Ballantine Books, 1986.

The Patient-Oriented Interview

2

The clinical interview is largely a function of collecting information. The details gathered enable the doctor to make accurate judgments and good clinical decisions. Cohen-Cole (1991) identifies three basic functions of the clinical interview: (1) gathering data to understand patients' problems, (2) developing rapport and responding to patients' emotions, and (3) educating patients and motivating them to adhere to management plans (Table 2.1). Optimal clinical care requires that each of these three areas be addressed.

History taking is part of the gathering of data. The "art" of history taking is often recognized by student interviewers who run into difficulty taking a case history, and observe an instructor who enters the examination room, knowing "just the right question" to ask the patient.

As students gain experience, they become more proficient in the content and flow of interviewing. Students will become more aware of content: what to ask, when to follow up with further questions, what follow-up questions are appropriate, and how to phrase their questions. As novice interviewers become experienced, the flow of the history improves greatly. Transitions between one part of the history and the next become more natural, and delivery of follow-up questions becomes natural and automatic.

The doctor can develop a doctor–patient rapport by recognizing and using the affective domain (the verbal or nonverbal "feeling" or emotional content of the interaction) to enhance the doctor's ability to gather information and gain the patient's cooperation.

Table 2.1 Functions of the clinical case history

1. Obtain information (ocular, medical, psychosocial)
2. Find out about a patient's problems and concerns
3. Understand the patient's context and environment so the doctor can best determine how to intervene (with testing, recommendations, and patient education)
4. Put the patient at ease in the clinical setting
5. Establish and build doctor–patient rapport
6. Set the tone for the examination (e.g., concerned, caring doctor; cooperative patient)
7. Start the clinical thinking and decision-making process (e.g., to think about what tests need to be done in the examination, and what initial diagnoses should be considered)

In the past, clinical care has often been very "doctor oriented." Doctors refer to complicated scientific terms and complex clinical procedures; emotional factors are not involved. The cognitive domain (facts and details) has traditionally been stressed in programs of clinical education.

To increase the success of the doctor–patient encounter, it has been shown that it is important to gear the doctor–patient interaction to the needs of the patient (Cohen-Cole 1991; Smith and Hoppe 1991; Levinson 1987; Anderson 1990; Beckman and Frankel 1984; Muldary 1983; Enelow and Swisher 1986; Okun 1992; Levenstein et al. 1989). The strategies outlined in this chapter stress the importance of the patient-centered interview.

COMPONENTS OF THE CLINICAL ENCOUNTER

The clinical examination is composed of three parts: the patient interview, the testing sequence, and the case disposition.

The patient interview consists of an introduction (in which the clinician greets the patient) and a case history (in which the clinician gathers information about the patient). Although the introduction is a very short component of the full visit, it is a crucial one. First impressions for both the doctor and the patient will form the foundation for the doctor–patient rapport. To set a positive tone, clinicians should introduce themselves by name and greet the patient by name. For example, "Good morning, Ms. Thompson. I'm Dr. Robertson and I'll be examining you today." A warm smile and handshake can also set a positive tone.

During the case history, the doctor gathers information about the patient's ocular status and general health. The testing sequence provides up-to-date ocular and clinical status. During the case disposition, the doctor discusses the results with the patient and works on developing a manage-

Table 2.2 Reasons for a "review of systems" approach

1. Patients may forget to mention something that was bothering them
2. Patients may assume that the doctor will be able to identify a problem, and would ask if it was important
3. Patients are sometimes afraid to look stupid and complain about something that is not important
4. Patients are sometimes afraid to ask about something that they think is serious
5. Patients sometimes think that a particular complaint is unimportant and not worth mentioning

ment plan with the patient. Communication at this point involves educating patients and building patient compliance (see Chapters 8 and 7, respectively). The case disposition should bring "closure" to the clinical encounter for both the doctor and the patient. Both individuals should feel satisfied when the doctor–patient encounter comes to an end.

THE CASE HISTORY

The case history generally starts with a general, open question such as: "How can I help you today?" or "What brings you in for an eye examination today?" The open-ended question allows patients to describe a chief complaint (or complaints) and to express, in their own words, how the problem affects their activities and function. Appropriate follow-up questions can be asked to elicit further information about the patient's complaints and symptoms. Open-ended questions give patients a nondirected opportunity to express complaints and to present their own perceptions of their problems, and also help strengthen the doctor–patient rapport.

Once the chief complaint and appropriate follow-up questions are covered sufficiently, the clinician moves to a series of other questions. In medicine, this is the part of the history referred to as the "review of systems" (Appendix B.7). This is a systematic approach with inquiries about all organ systems and functions to identify any underlying problems that might have been missed in the earlier discussion. Since patients do not always express when they have a problem, or they may forget to mention a symptom, it is important to be able to rule out any problems that have not been mentioned (Table 2.2).

Optometric Case History

The eye doctor also asks a series of questions covering a full range of ocular functions and symptoms (see Primary Care Optometric Interview, Appendix B.1). It is important to ask all of the questions to make sure that the patient has not omitted anything significant. The optometric case history includes the following areas of inquiry:

Chief complaint

Current ocular status and visual demands

Patient ocular history

Patient medical history

Family ocular history

Family medical history

Follow-up questions should include the following categories: severity, onset, quality, location, duration, frequency, change, associated factors, history, and "modifying factors" (see Follow-up Questions on Symptoms, Appendix B.2). Inquiring about whether the patient has had a history of the problem can enlighten the doctor on previous therapies. "Modifying factors" describe conditions that make the symptom better and worse. It is often helpful to know the factors that intensify and remedy a situation to understand the potential cause.

Case history questions can be catered for visits related to specific problems. Sample case history questions specific to contact lenses (Appendix B.3), vision therapy (Appendix B.4), low vision (Appendix B.5), and pediatrics (Appendix B.6) are provided.

Information to Gather

Information that the clinician should collect during the case history falls across two categories: the cognitive domain and the affective domain.

The cognitive content of a message includes the facts and details provided verbally by the patient. The cognitive content has traditionally been stressed in programs of clinical education. Does the patient have any symptoms of blurred vision? Any eyepain? Any flashes or floaters? The cognitive level relies on the patient's thought processes, knowledge, and reasoning. Emotional factors are not involved in this level of communication.

The affective domain, on the other hand, refers to the "feeling" or emotional content of the interaction. The affective content can be verbal or nonverbal. Patients may state their feelings, emotions, or attitudes verbally. More often, these components are expressed subtly, and the doctor has to be very observant to notice these messages. Patients present to clinical examinations with a variety of emotions. These emotions and the doctor's response (or lack of response) can affect the doctor's ability to gather clinical information and gain the patient's cooperation.

Muldary (1983) indicates that messages are composed of cognitive message units and affective message units. Both content and feelings give meaning to a message. Ignoring or overlooking either aspect prevents the listener from understanding the full meaning of a speaker's communication.

Some messages are basically cognitive, with some affective undertones, and some are predominantly affective. In addition to recognizing the meaning transmitted by both domains, it is helpful to perceive the balance within a message. Patients sometimes stay within the cognitive domain, with subtle emotional expressions. When a patient makes a strongly affective communication, however, the doctor who recognizes this can be very effective by responding appropriately. Strongly affective comments are answered most effectively with responses that are highly affective. The following scenario presents two different ways of responding to an affective statement. Which of the two doctors demonstrates a more effective response?

A 36-year-old patient is learning to insert and remove contact lenses. The patient has never worn contact lenses before. Insertion and removal are practiced so the patient can take the lenses home.

PATIENT: I am really afraid to put these contact lenses into my eyes.

DOCTOR: I can see that you are feeling uncomfortable about this. Many patients who are learning to insert and remove their lenses feel uncomfortable in the beginning. It usually becomes easier as you practice; for many patients, it eventually becomes second nature. We'll go slowly, and I'll show you exactly what to do. If you have any questions, or if you need to take a break, just let me know.

DOCTOR: That's why I'm going to show you how to insert your lenses. You put the lens at the edge of your index finger, you hold your lids open with your other fingers. Then you just put the lens in. To take the lenses out, you hold the lids with your fingers again, you move the lens over to the white part of your eye, and you pinch the lens out between your thumb and index finger.

In the first scenario, the doctor responded to the patient's highly affective comment, reassuring the patient that fear is not unusual, and that insertion and removal get easier with practice. Like the patient's comment in this scenario, the doctor's response is also strongly affective.

In the second scenario, although the patient's comment is affective, the doctor's response is highly cognitive. The doctor gives the patient useful information about the process of insertion and removal, but it does not appear to be at a time when the patient is receptive to learning. (More information on patient education will be covered in Chapter 8.)

The doctor who stays only at the cognitive level during the case history misses a lot of information. The doctor who is skilled in "reading" a patient's feelings and concerns can often pick up signs that will help care for the patient.

A 62-year-old woman has age-related macular degeneration, first diagnosed three years ago. She presents to the doctor complaining of blurred vision. Although the condition has remained a dry form of macular degeneration, the patient has noticed some changes in clarity over time.

PATIENT: The blurred vision that I have had over the last few years has made it harder and harder for me to function at work. I feel like I'm losing control, and I can't handle it anymore. (Patient is speaking at an affective level, and expresses frustration with the progressive decrease in vision.)

DOCTOR: The visual problem that you have, age-related macular degeneration, frequently occurs with a progressive decrease in vision over time. (The doctor responds at a cognitive level, giving the patient more information about the diagnosis.)

DOCTOR: I can understand your frustration about your blurred vision. It must be very difficult to try to work, when you are having trouble seeing. Patients with the same problem that you have sometimes report that their vision changes, but one of the things that I am going to do today is to see if there is anything that I can do to improve your vision. If you have any questions for me as we go along, please feel free to ask me. (The doctor responds to the patient's concern on an affective level, and reassures the patient that an attempt will be made to improve the patient's ability to function. Finally, identifying the patient's fear and concern, the doctor invites the patient to ask any questions that arise.)

In which of the two scenarios do you think the patient would be most comfortable and ready to participate in the rest of the examination? In both cases, the doctor gives the patient a little further information about the diagnosis and the fact that changes in vision over time are not unusual.

In the first scenario, the doctor gives the patient further information about the diagnosis, but does nothing to address the patient's concerns. In the second scenario, the doctor responds to the patient's concerns by conveying awareness of the difficulties, and by reassuring the patient that the problem will be investigated during the examination.

Patients who present to clinical settings with strong emotional feelings are often labeled "difficult" patients by health care workers who find it challenging to work with these patients. Often, what they need is acknowledgment of their emotional concerns so they know that the doctor is listening. A special section on dealing with "difficult patients" will be covered in Chapter 14. By attending to the patient's emotional cues in addition to the factual content, the doctor can make the clinical encounter a much more pleasant and reassuring experience.

TYPES OF QUESTIONS AND STATEMENTS

In the clinical environment, *what* you say to the patient is as important as *how* you say it. Asking a question effectively may elicit a more comprehensive and clinically useful response. Communicating effectively can improve a doctor's ability to address a patient's needs.

In the following section, a variety of types of questions and statements will be discussed to enable the doctor to consider how the required information is obtained during the clinical interview. Communicating with patients is often a matter of style. A wide range of questions and statements can be utilized in the clinical interview (Table 2.3).

Open-Ended vs. Closed-Ended Questions

Open-Ended Questions

Open-ended questions are unstructured, undirected ways of allowing responders to choose their own focus and perspective in providing an answer. Open-ended questions cannot be answered solely by "yes" or "no" and they typically start with one of the following: "What," "How," "When," "Where," and "Why," which generally require more than a one- or two-word answer. This type of question allows speakers to convey information about their attitudes, values, and feelings; closed-ended questions generally do not provide this insight.

An open-ended question is typically used at the very beginning of the case history to start the interview. Open-ended questions are used to bring up new topics as the case history proceeds. Follow-up questions become more specific to allow the doctor to obtain particular details.

Examples:

How can I help you today?

What brings you in for an eye examination today?

What activities make your eyes feel tired?

What symptoms do you experience when you use your computer?

When do your eyes become red and irritated?

Table 2.3 Types of questions and statements

Open-ended vs. closed-ended questions
Direct vs. indirect questions
Compound questions
Leading questions
Laundry list questions
Informing questions/statements
Facilitative questions/statements
Clarifying questions/statements
Reflection
Paraphrasing
Checking
Summarizing
Validating questions/statements
Acknowledging questions/statements
Confronting questions/statements

How is your general health?

What visual activities do you do at work?

Closed-Ended Questions

Closed-ended questions are very structured questions that can be answered by "yes," "no," or by just a few words.

Examples:

Do you see well with your current reading glasses?

Do you get headaches?

Do you wear contact lenses?

Do you have glaucoma?

Does anyone in your family have glaucoma?

Are you taking any medications?

How old are you?

By choosing open-ended or closed-ended questions, the questioner sets the stage for the form of the answer: a lengthier, broader answer in the case of the open-ended question or a single-word response in the case of the closed-ended question.

Open-ended questions are generally considered preferable for opening up new areas of inquiry. Closed-ended ones are more useful for seeking specific details. As interviewers move from general to specific in clinical case histories, they generally move from open-ended to closed-ended questions.

As part of "knowing your audience," the doctor should consider whether open- or closed-ended questions are preferable for specific types of patients. "Rambling" patients tend to do better with closed-ended questions, which help to narrow their responses. "Quiet" patients often respond better to open-ended questions, which encourage them to communicate actively with the doctor. These and other types of difficult patients will be discussed in detail in Chapter 14.

Case history questions usually go from general to more specific; as they do, questions very often change from open-ended to closed-ended forms.

DR. RICHARDS: Mr. Clarren, what brings you in for an eye examination today? (The doctor starts the examination with a very broad, open-ended question.)

MR. CLARREN: I've been having headaches. Real bad headaches.

DR. RICHARDS: When do you experience the headaches? (Still an open-ended question, but now it is more specific, because it relates specifically to the headaches.)

MR. CLARREN: I get them after I've been reading for awhile.

DR. RICHARDS: How long do you have to be reading to experience the headaches? (The line of questioning becomes narrower, with specific questions about the headaches.)

MR. CLARREN: They seem to start about 45 minutes after I start to read. I used to be able to read longer, but now it's 45 minutes, and that's my limit.

DR. RICHARDS: What do the headaches feel like? (The doctor works to establish severity, quality, and location.)

MR. CLARREN: I get a throbbing sensation right here. (Patient points frontally.) It gets pretty bad. Sometimes it's really uncomfortable.

DR. RICHARDS: What do you do when you get the headaches?

MR. CLARREN: I stop reading, and I take an aspirin.

DR. RICHARDS: Do these help? (A closed-ended question.)

MR. CLARREN: Yes, it makes it much better.

DR. RICHARDS: How long have you been having these headaches?

MR. CLARREN: About three months.

DR. RICHARDS: Have they changed at all, over time?

MR. CLARREN: They're getting slightly worse.

DR. RICHARDS: How often do you get the headaches?

MR. CLARREN: About two to three times a week. Sometimes a little more often.

DR. RICHARDS: Are there any other problems that you're having with your vision? (Having gathered adequate information about the patient's headaches, the doctor now asks a general question to elicit any other complaints.)

Direct versus Indirect Questions

Direct Questions

Direct questions are specific questions that leave little doubt about what information is being requested. Direct questions can be open-ended or closed-ended, depending on the type of response elicited by the form of the question.

Direct Open-Ended Question: What type of activities do you do at work?

Direct Closed-Ended Question: Are you currently working?

Indirect Questions

Indirect questions do not sound like questions, but they elicit information. Unlike traditional open-ended questions, indirect questions generally do not appear, or sound, like questions.

Indirect Question: It sounds like you had a lot of problems with your health when you were a child. You must have spent a lot of time at the doctor's office.

Indirect Question: You mentioned that your vision has been getting poorer and poorer over the last few years. That must be very stressful.

Compound Questions

Compound questions present the respondent with multiple questions at the same time. The compound question is not an effective type of question because it frequently leaves the respondent confused or uncertain about how to respond. Consider the following example:

DOCTOR: Do you ever get headaches or see double?

What if the patient gets headaches, but does not see double? Should the patient say "yes" or "no," and how will the questioner know which question is being answered? What if the patient sees double, but does not get headaches? Again, the patient is faced with a dilemma.

Compound inquiries should be avoided, because they are confusing and ambiguous. When multiple questions need to be asked, they should be asked separately.

Leading Questions

Leading questions give the patient a suggested answer to the question.

Leading Question: When I put this lens in front of your eye, does it make the letters clearer? (The patient is prompted to think that the lens should make the letter clearer, and is encouraged to answer "yes."

Neutral Question: What happens when I put this lens in front of your eye? (This form leaves the patient with the responsibility of telling what happens with the lens.)

Leading Question: You don't get any headaches, do you? (This sets the patient up for a "no" response.)

Neutral Question: Do you ever experience headaches? (This gives the patient the opportunity to provide the appropriate response.)

Laundry List Questions

Laundry list questions present the respondent with a set of possible responses:

Do you get the double vision every day, once a week, twice a week, or a few times a month?

The disadvantage of laundry list questions is that respondents often feel that they must answer with one of the choices presented. If their true answer is not one of the choices, they may not respond appropriately.

Although "laundry list" questions are not optimal forms of questioning, there are times when these questions can be useful. For "quiet" patients who are very reserved, the "laundry list" may make them feel reassured and less intimidated because they are presented with choices.

When using "laundry list" questions for specific purposes, it is best to end the question with a choice that goes beyond the range of the other answers:

Do you get double vision every day, once a week, twice a week, or some other frequency? (This way, the patient can answer with a response other than those listed.)

Informing Questions and Statements

Informing questions and statements are verbal communications that are used either to seek factual and objective information from a respondent (informing questions) or to provide factual and objective information to an individual (informing comments).

Informing Statements

Informing statements are frequently used at the end of the examination, for patient education purposes, to share information about a patient's diagnosis.

> Informing Statement: Mr. Rodriguez, my examination today indicates that you are nearsighted. That means that you see near objects better than you see objects at a distance, and that you need to wear glasses for distance.

> Informing Statement: Ms. O'Hara, I examined you today to determine what is causing your blurred vision. What I found is that you have early signs of cataracts. This means that one of the structures in your eye, the lens, is starting to become less transparent. The good news about this is that you don't have to do anything about this at the current time, and I will monitor your progress over time to see if any changes occur.

When using informing statements, it is important not to appear to lecture, proselytize, or preach, since these actions can make patients uncomfortable. The goal of informing should be to present the facts and provide information objectively and respectfully.

Informing statements are frequently followed by clarifying questions and statements (see below) to see if the patient has understood what has been said.

Informing Questions

Informing questions are most commonly used when the health care professional asks the patient about specific information during the case history. These questions may at first be fairly broad, and become more specific as more information is gathered. With a set of consecutive informing questions, the health professional can probe the patient to obtain more information about a particular symptom or problem. When the health professional uses these questions to obtain further information at a greater depth of understanding, they are often referred to as probing questions.

In the case below, which includes part of a case history on a 38-year-old patient, each of the doctor's questions is an informing inquiry.

> DOCTOR: Ms. Marchesi, do you ever experience blurred vision at near distances?

> PATIENT: Yes, when I have been reading I sometimes notice that my vision gets blurry.

> DOCTOR: Does your vision get blurred as soon as you start reading, or does it become blurry after you have been reading for awhile?

> PATIENT: It doesn't get blurry until after I have been reading for awhile. I'll be doing fine, and then all of a sudden the letters just start to get blurry.

> DOCTOR: About how long do you have to be reading for this to happen?

PATIENT: It doesn't happen until I have been reading for about an hour. Then I start to get the blurring, and I have to stop reading.

DOCTOR: Do you get any other symptoms with the blurring?

PATIENT: Yes, sometimes I get headaches when it happens, and sometimes my eyes get watery and they feel really tired.

The doctor can continue to probe the patient until all relevant information has been obtained.

Facilitative Questions and Statements

Facilitation involves any verbal or nonverbal communication that encourages the respondent to speak further. Examples are phrases such as "Keep going" and "Tell me more about that"; an affirmative head nod; and attentive silence, in which the speaker is free to continue. Good listeners are skillful at using facilitative behaviors. These techniques will be discussed in greater detail in Chapter 3 (pp. 41–52). Table 3.1 shows a wide array of facilitative statements and actions.

Clarifying Questions and Statements

Clarification enables interviewers to confirm what they think they have heard and identify any misunderstandings in information that has been gathered. There are four common types of clarifying statements: reflection, paraphrasing, checking, and summarizing.

Reflection

The interviewer "reflects" a patient's response by actually repeating some of the patient's words. In addition to clarifying, this encourages the speaker to continue and develop the same line of thought.

PATIENT: I'm very worried about the symptoms that I have been experiencing.

DOCTOR: Very worried about the symptoms? (This encourages the patient to go on and discuss the problem in further detail.)

PATIENT: My eyes feel very dry in the morning.

DOCTOR: Very dry? (This encourages the patient to go on and elaborate on the symptom of dryness.)

Paraphrasing

As with reflection, paraphrasing allows the interviewer to repeat the essence of a patient's statement. Paraphrasing is actually at a different level because in paraphrasing, interviewers recapitulate what they have heard in their own words. Since the doctor is not just repeating the patient's words, but interpreting the message and putting it into his or her own words, this is a higher level than reflection. Paraphrasing is a good technique to verify understanding.

> DOCTOR: So, my understanding is that you experience headaches and blurry vision only at near after you have been reading for about an hour. Until then, everything is nice and clear. Is that correct?

Checking

Checking has been called the "most important information-gathering skill" and the one that is "least utilized" (Cohen-Cole 1991).

The complexity of language often results in misinterpretations and misunderstandings. By checking, the doctor can confirm that what is understood is what the patient really meant. (Remember from Chapter 1 that the message heard is not always the same as the message that was sent.) Checking facilitates correction and clarification by the patient. It also shows that the doctor is interested in what the patient is saying. In addition to the advantage of clarifying the content of the message, patients often find checking reassuring because it tells them that the doctor has an accurate understanding of their concerns and personal information.

> Ms. Weinstein, I'd like to check briefly with you to make sure that I understand what you told me about your decrease in vision. You said that it happened suddenly, that only your right eye was affected, that there was no pain associated with it, and that your vision returned fully after about five minutes. Is that correct?

Summarizing

In summarizing, the doctor presents a brief review of what has been understood of the main points of a patient's communication. The patient can then clarify any misinterpretation in the doctor's understanding.

> Mr. Lawrence, I understand that you are experiencing blurred vision and headaches when you read, but that you have no problems at distance.

Validating Questions and Statements

Like clarifying questions and statements, validation helps to confirm meaning and accuracy. Validation actually goes a step further because it involves interpretation of nonverbal cues in addition to the verbal statement.

Validation requires a listener to be a good observer and an astute listener. Legitimation is a form of validation that communicates an acceptance and recognition (validation) of the patient's emotional experience

(Cohen-Cole 1991). Legitimation does not mean that the health care professional necessarily agrees with the patient's view or response. It shows that the interviewer has enough respect for the patient to listen and understand the patient's point of view. For many people, legitimation can be a particularly effective technique of communication. Legitimation can be particularly helpful in dealing with some "difficult" types of patients, such as patients who are angry, anxious, or uncooperative (see Chapter 14).

> Mr. Louis, you appear apprehensive about using drops in your eyes, even though they are itching and bothering you.

> Ms. Kipnis, you still seem worried about the recent change in your prescription. We can discuss any further questions or concerns that are still on your mind.

Acknowledging Statements

Acknowledging statements are similar to validating statements, except that acknowledging statements emphasize the response along the affective dimensions. Emotions and feelings can sometimes be an obstacle to the communication process if unacknowledged by the listener. The acknowledging statement is a helpful technique for a variety of "difficult" patient encounters (see Chapter 14).

Ignoring a patient's emotions and feelings can make a doctor appear insensitive and unobservant. Acknowledging a patient's emotions, even when they are negative, can be helpful in getting the patient to address her emotions.

> You appear a little bit nervous today, Ms. Hoff. Is there anything I can do to make you feel more comfortable?

Confronting Questions and Statements

Confronting questions and statements are used to approach a patient very directly. These questions are sometimes useful in dealing with "difficult patients" and patients who are potential alcoholics, drug abusers, or victims of domestic abuse (see Chapters 13 and 14). Interviewers usually do not use this technique unless they have tried to handle the subject with less severe techniques; however, confrontation is sometimes the only way to get respondents to address topics that they have been avoiding.

> Confronting Statement: "Ms. Marcus, you sound very angry. We have to talk about this now, so we can continue with your examination."

On the surface, confronting statements may sometimes look like acknowledging or validating statements, but what often makes them different are the nonverbal and paralanguage cues that accompany them. Confronting statements are usually delivered in a very firm voice, with a stern facial expression.

Since confronting questions on these topics are frequently sharp and painful, and they often elicit emotional responses, the health professional may sometimes choose to defer confronting questions of this nature until the required clinical information has been gathered and the patient is not uncomfortable or on edge.

COMMUNICATION PATTERNS IN THE CLINICAL INTERVIEW

Doctors use questions during the clinical interview to elicit information. In addition to the particular types of questions discussed in the previous section, the sequence and patterns of questions affect the clinical interview (Figure 2.1).

The Funnel Approach

The funnel approach begins with a broad, open-ended question and the line of questioning narrows as the conversation proceeds (Figure 2.1a).

DOCTOR: What brings you in today? (Open-ended question.)

PATIENT: I am finding that my vision is blurry.

DOCTOR: What types of activities are you doing when you find that your vision is blurry? (Still open-ended, but narrower because it relates specifically to the blurry vision.)

PATIENT: Usually reading and writing. Anything at near is difficult.

DOCTOR: How long has your vision at near been blurry? (The questioning is becoming narrower.)

PATIENT: For about the past three months.

DOCTOR: Is your vision at near better when you wear your glasses? (A closed-ended question.)

PATIENT: Yes, but it's not as good as it used to be.

The Inverted Funnel Approach

The inverted funnel approach starts with a closed-ended question and gradually moves toward broad, open questions (Figure 2.1b).

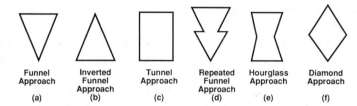

Figure 2.1 Interview approaches. The sequence of questions in an interview can be described by the patterns that they create. Six interviewing styles are illustrated. (a) The funnel approach begins with a broad, open-ended question, and gradually moves toward closed-ended questions that gather more specific, detailed information. (b) The inverted funnel approach starts with a closed-ended question, and gradually moves toward broad, open-ended questions. (c) The tunnel approach involves a sequence of questions, all of which are a common form or depth. A tunnel sequence may be a series of open, or closed, questions. (d) The repeated funnel approach involves a series of back-to-back funnel sequences. It is often helpful to use a repeated funnel approach going from one topic to another during the case history. For each new topic, the question starts out broad; the questions become more specific as information is collected. As the next topic is started, a broad question is used to open the line of questioning. (e) The hourglass approach involves a "broad–narrow–broad" sequence that goes from open-ended questions to closed-ended questions, and then back to open-ended inquiries. (f) The diamond approach involves a "narrow–broad–narrow" sequence that goes from closed-ended questions to open-ended questions, and then back to closed-ended inquiries.

DOCTOR: Do you ever experience blurry vision? (A closed-ended question.)

PATIENT: Yes.

DOCTOR: Is your vision blurry at distance or near? (Another narrow, restricted question.)

PATIENT: It's blurry at near.

DOCTOR: Do you have any other symptoms when you do near work? (The questions are becoming more open, allowing the patient greater opportunity for expression.)

PATIENT: My eyes get tired sometimes.

DOCTOR: What other types of problems have you noticed with your vision? (The inverted funnel approach concludes with an open-ended question.)

PATIENT: My eyes also get red and irritated sometimes, especially at the end of a long, hard day.

The inverted funnel approach often works best with the patient who is "nervous," and who may be intimidated by broad questions early in the interview. Once the patient becomes more relaxed, the doctor can proceed to broader questions. If the doctor needs to return to narrower questions later in the interview, the conversation may take the form of a diamond (Figure 2.1f).

The Tunnel Approach

The tunnel approach involves a sequence of questions, all of which are a common form or depth (Figure 2.1c). The tunnel may be a sequence of open or closed questions.

> DOCTOR: Do you experience any headaches? (Closed-ended, requires yes/no response.)
>
> PATIENT: No.
>
> DOCTOR: Do you ever notice any flashes of light? (Closed-ended, requires yes/no response.)
>
> PATIENT: No.
>
> DOCTOR: Do your eyes ever itch? (Closed-ended, requires yes/no response.)
>
> PATIENT: No.
>
> DOCTOR: Do your eyes ever tear? (Closed-ended, requires yes/no response.)

The Repeated Funnel Approach

Clinical interviews are generally described as going from open to closed. Interviewers frequently begin with a general statement ("What brings you in today?") and narrow the topic of discussion to gather more information. This is similar to the funnel approach.

Many interviews actually take the form of a repeated funnel, in which a general question leads to more specific questions on a particular topic; then, another general question leads to more specific questions on another topic (Figure 2.1d).

> DOCTOR: What brings you in today? (Open-ended question.)
>
> PATIENT: I am finding that my vision is blurry.
>
> DOCTOR: What activities are you doing when your vision is blurry? (Still open-ended, but narrower because it relates specifically to the blurry vision.)
>
> PATIENT: Usually reading and writing. Anything at near is difficult.
>
> DOCTOR: How long has your vision at near been blurry? (The questioning is becoming narrower.)
>
> PATIENT: For about the past three months.
>
> DOCTOR: Is your vision at near better when you wear your glasses? (A closed-ended question.)

PATIENT: Yes, but it's not as good as it used to be.

DOCTOR: What other types of symptoms have you experienced with your vision? (An open-ended question opens the way for another topic.)

PATIENT: I notice that I get headaches when I'm reading.

DOCTOR: Tell me about the headaches that you have been experiencing. (Still open-ended, but more specific because it relates to the headaches.)

PATIENT: It's a dull, throbbing pain, right at the front of my forehead.

DOCTOR: How long have you been experiencing the headaches? (The questions are becoming narrower, now.)

PATIENT: About two months.

DOCTOR: Have the headaches changed in intensity over time? (Another narrow question.)

PATIENT: Yes, they seem to be getting worse.

Once a symptom is elicited, and some general information is obtained about the problem, a series of follow-up questions investigates severity, onset, quality, location, duration, frequency, and other factors. This sequence often uses a tunnel approach. Many of these questions are similar in form and gather information of comparable depth.

The Hourglass Approach

The hourglass approach takes a broad–narrow–broad form (Figure 2.1e). This approach sometimes emerges with the "silent" patient who is not identified as "quiet" at the onset of the interview. Many doctors open the interview with a general, open question (broad). "Silent" patients often do not respond well to this type of question, and doctors find the information difficult to ascertain. When they recognize that the patient is "silent" they go to a narrower approach, to make the patient more comfortable. Once the patient is participating to a greater extent, they can then return to a broader approach and obtain additional required information.

The hourglass approach may also work well with patients who are very verbal and need to express themselves. This patient may prefer open-ended questions at the beginning of the interview, but the doctor may then need to narrow down the discussion to get specific details. It may make these patients more satisfied if the discussion is widened again at the end to give them an opportunity to fully express their feelings. Histrionic and narcissistic patients may benefit from this strategy (see Chapter 15).

In general, if the interviewer is at an impasse and is not getting responses to his questions, it is often helpful to change the form of questioning. Sometimes by asking the same question in a different way, the doctor can acquire the necessary information.

HIDDEN AGENDA

Patients do not always come in to the doctor and say what is on their minds. They sometimes keep their motivations for making the appointment to themselves until the doctor picks up a cue for a hidden agenda (Barsky 1981).

Sometimes patients are embarrassed to ask what is on their mind, sometimes they are afraid to ask, and sometimes they are afraid to look stupid. In any case, the patient is concerned about something. The skillful interviewer is perceptive in picking up these hidden—but very realistic—concerns.

Hidden agendas often become apparent during the testing sequence or near the end of the examination. They are a reminder that the interview does not end at the completion of the case history.

A 42-year-old female, presents for an examination. The case history is completed, and the doctor is almost finished with the testing sequence.

MS. COOPER: Doctor, are you going to do a glaucoma test on me?

DOCTOR: Yes, I am going to do one in just a few minutes. Why do you ask—do you have any particular concerns about having glaucoma? (Doctor picks up on and immediately addresses the patient's concern.)

MS. COOPER: My brother had an eye examination last week and they found out that he has glaucoma; I was concerned about whether I may have it, too.

DOCTOR: I'm glad you told me about that. I am definitely going to do a glaucoma test on you toward the end of the examination. Your pressures have always been normal since you have been coming to me, and they were normal when I saw you last year. But pressures can change over time, so it's important to check them. I'm glad you discussed your concern with me. When I do the test in a few minutes, I will discuss my result with you, and I'll be happy to answer any questions that you have.

MS. COOPER: Great—it certainly will be a relief to know how I am doing.

THE PATIENT-ORIENTED INTERVIEW:
INFORMATION THAT SHOULD BE GATHERED

Many people think that the case history should primarily be a collection of information about a patient's symptoms and medical history. This view ignores a number of other factors that contribute to a patient's health and that affect the patient's ability to deal with disease and illness.

When conducting the case history, the interviewer should take note of the following areas:

1. Ocular/medical status
2. Psychological/emotional status
3. Environmental/occupational conditions
4. Sociological factors
5. Cultural factors
6. Patient's health beliefs

TRANSITION FROM HISTORY TO EXAMINATION SEQUENCE

Skillful interviewers are able to make a smooth transition from the end of the case history to the start of the examination sequence. Transitions are a matter of style and can be handled in different ways.

One effective way of handling the transition is to summarize the patient's concerns expressed during the case history. This shows patients that you have heard their concerns and reassures them that you are planning to address them and make observations during your examination. Finally, it allows the patient to correct any misconceptions or misunderstandings about information that has been gathered so far.

An abrupt, unexplained change can put a patient on edge; a smooth transition can reassure the patient that the problems expressed were clearly understood.

QUESTIONS FOR THOUGHT

1. Discuss the functions of the clinical interview. How do you accomplish these functions during the interview?
2. In a clinical case history, what is the difference in gathering information in the cognitive and affective domains? To be a good clinician, does the health care professional have to attend to information in both domains? Can a clinician be as effective by collecting information in the cognitive domain, without attending to the affective domain?
3. Give two examples of each of the following types of questions.
   a. open-ended question
   b. closed-ended question
   c. compound question
   d. laundry list question
   e. leading question
   f. neutral question

   g. clarifying question

   h. confronting question

4. If a patient expresses a "hidden agenda" toward the end of the clinical examination, does that mean that the doctor did not do a good job of eliciting the patient's problems or concerns at the beginning of the examination?

5. In this chapter it is stated that the case disposition should bring "closure" to the clinical encounter for both the doctor and patient. Patients will probably be satisfied if the doctor can solve their problems in a caring manner. What does the doctor look for in "closure" to the doctor–patient encounter? What makes you feel that you have done a good job at the end of a clinical encounter?

6. Observe a clinical examination and use the sheet provided in Appendix A to record your observations. (You can either observe a colleague's examination or videotape an examination that you perform and make observations as you watch the videotape.) Fill out the checklist and answer the questions, as directed.

7. You are conducting a case history and experience the following interactions with patients. (For each statement provided, a brief patient background is given.) Provide effective responses for each of the following statements.

   a. "My vision keeps getting worse and worse over the years. How much worse is it going to get?" (This patient is a 72-year-old female, with age-related macular degeneration.)

   b. "I don't have the time to go to the doctor again for another test. I can't keep taking off from work because my boss gets angry." (This patient is a 52-year-old male, and you are referring him for a fluorescein angiogram as a result of diabetic retinopathy.)

   c. "I know that I want contact lenses, but I don't think that I'll ever be able to put them in my eyes. I hate wearing my glasses, but the thought of putting something in my eyes really bothers me." (This patient is a 32-year-old female who presented to your office because she is interested in getting contact lenses. When you begin to fit her, she expresses concern and discomfort about putting lenses in her eyes.)

   d. "Why do you want me to come back for additional tests? Doctors are always looking for ways to make more money." (This patient is a 47-year-old female whom you have examined for the first time. You found that she has moderately elevated intraocular pressures, and you have just explained that you want her to return to your office for visual field testing and a recheck of her intraocular pressures.)

   e. "Why are you asking me all of these questions? You're the doctor, and you should be able to tell me if there are any problems with my eyes." (This patient is a 62-year-old male who has presented to your office for the first time. You are doing a case history, and he shows some resistance in responding to your questions.)

REFERENCES

Anderson CA. Patient Teaching and Communicating in an Information Age. Albany, NY: Delmar Publishers, 1990.

Barsky AJ. Hidden reasons some patients visit doctors. Annals of Internal Medicine 94:492–498, 1981.

Beckman HB, Frankel RM. The effect of physician behavior on the collection of data. Annals of Internal Medicine 101:692–696, 1984.

Cohen-Cole SA. The Medical Interview: The Three-Function Approach. St. Louis: Mosby Year Book, 1991.

Enelow AJ, Swisher SN. Interviewing and Patient Care. New York: Oxford University Press, 1986.

Levinson D. A Guide to the Clinical Interview. Philadelphia: W.B. Saunders, 1987.

Levenstein JH, et al. Patient-centered clinical interviewing. In: Stewart M, Roter D, eds., Communicating with Medical Patients. Newbury Park, CA: Sage Publications, 1989.

Muldary TW. Interpersonal Relations for Health Professionals—A Social Skills Approach. New York: Macmillan, 1983.

Okun BF. Effective Helping Interviewing and Counseling Techniques. Pacific Grove, CA: Brooks/Cole, 1992.

Smith RC, Hoppe RB. The patient's story: Integrating the patient- and physician-centered approaches to interviewing. Annals of Internal Medicine 115:470–477, 1991.

ADDITIONAL READINGS

Cassell EJ. Talking with Patients (Vols. 1 and 2). Cambridge, MA: MIT Press, 1985.

Cassell EJ. The Nature of Suffering. New York: Oxford University Press, 1991.

Donnelly WJ. Righting the medical record—Transforming chronicle into story. Journal of the American Medical Association 260:823–825, 1988.

Fischer BA. Fine-tuning the message. Optometric Economics 2:13–21, 1992.

Frankel R, Beckman H. Evaluating the patient's primary problem(s). In Stewart M, Roter D, eds., Communicating with Medical Patients. London: Sage Publications, 1989: 86–98.

Pearson JC, Nelson PE. Understanding and Sharing—An Introduction to Speech Communication. Dubuque, IA: William C. Brown, 1988.

Stewart CJ, Cash WB. Interviewing Principles and Practices. Dubuque, IA: William C. Brown, 1988.

3

Good Listening and Responding Skills

Communication does not involve only the spoken word. An essential component of good communication is listening to the speaker attentively. Good listeners are good communicators.

It has been estimated that in 80% of our waking hours, we are involved in some form of communication (Pryor 1987). Of those hours:

9% is spent writing,

16% is spent reading,

30% is spent speaking, and

45% is spent listening.

Standard education emphasizes training in reading and writing skills. With the amount of time spent listening (almost 50%), it is surprising that so little attention is paid to developing good listening skills.

Listening is imperative in the clinical environment. The clinical interviewer must hear the patient's symptoms, complaints, and concerns and must understand what they are, and how they affect the patient. It would be difficult, if not impossible, to provide ethical care without listening to the patient's concerns and desires.

Studies suggest that doctors talk more than they listen (Levinson 1987). Beckman and Frankel (1984) found that in 69% of patient interviews, physicians interrupted their patients within the first 18 seconds of the clinical encounter. In 77% of the interviews, patients' reasons for presenting to the doctor were never fully explained during the interview. Korsch and Negrete (1972) found that a significant proportion of mothers were not given an opportunity to express their chief concerns for bringing their children for pediatric examinations. Obstacles to listening can result in an incomplete collection of patient information and an inaccurate representation of patient problems.

Just as we differentiate vision and sight in eye care (sight is the reception of light waves at the eye; vision is the perception and interpretation of visual stimuli), so too must hearing and listening be differentiated (hearing is the reception of sound waves at the ear; listening is the perception and interpretation of sounds). Good listening is an active process. Active listening involves processing the verbal message, observing the nonverbal cues, and integrating both. Becoming a better listener or "receiver" involves concentrating on details, staying attentive, and encouraging the speaker to continue.

By demonstrating active listening, the doctor conveys signs of sensitivity, interest, and concern to the patient. This can facilitate further discussion. Aside from encouraging the patient to share valuable information, good listening also contributes to the development of good doctor–patient rapport.

Clinical training programs emphasize teaching students to learn to use pieces of equipment and to perform various procedures. In previous years, clinical programs have rarely addressed listening to patients. This chapter provides recommendations on improving listening skills with patients.

OBSTACLES TO LISTENING

Barriers to effective listening, or noise, as discussed in Chapter 1, include loss of concentration, lack of interest in the patient's story, biases and prejudices, environmental obstacles, and premature conclusions.

Loss of concentration and the "mind wandering" phenomenon are common causes of poor listening. Why does the mind tend to wander? Lucas (1989) suggests that although people can talk at 125–150 words a minute, the brain can actually process 400–800 words a minute. The difference between use and capability leaves the brain with a lot of spare "brain time," in which the mind can wander to something else. Good listeners, however, use this lag to review what has been discussed, to take in nonverbal cues, and to interpret the meaning. By concentrating on what is said, and making sure one's mind is not wandering, the listener can focus attention on the speaker. It is helpful to monitor your listening from time to time to make sure that you are still concentrating on the patient.

Poor listening attitudes and lack of interest in the patient's situation constitute another type of barrier. We may sometimes think that what the patient is about to say is not important. Many listeners let their personal biases and prejudices affect their listening. Environmental obstacles ("noise") are also barriers to good listening. Loud background noises and other distractions within the environment can interfere with listening.

Jumping to conclusions is also a common aspect of poor listening. We sometimes make our own conclusions before the patient has even finished speaking. When we form an initial conclusion, we may then tend to ignore subsequent details that are not consistent with our impressions. It is important to keep an open mind in communications, not to hear just what we want to hear, but to hear what the patient wants to tell us.

LISTENING ACTIVELY

A good listening attitude involves a *genuine interest* in patients and their concerns. Eye contact and an open, positive attitude are also aspects of active listening.

Physically attending to a speaker is also an essential part of active listening. It is generally recommended that the doctor face the patient directly, so the axis of the doctor's shoulders is parallel to the axis of the patient's shoulders (Figure 3.1). This is generally referred to as facing the patient *squarely*. Doctors who are facing the patient at a different angle may be perceived as uninterested or inattentive. Doctors who avoid eye contact may be perceived in the same way (Chapter 4, pp. 55–56). Eye contact is an important part of demonstrating one's capacity to be a good listener.

A *forward lean* of the upper body also conveys a receptiveness toward the speaker. Body posture, eye contact, and a forward lean demonstrate a physical orientation to the speaker.

In listening, the listener's attitude, facial expressions, mannerisms, and gestures can also convey good listening skills. It is helpful for the doctor to appear physically and emotionally relaxed and at ease during the examination to help put the patient at ease. A doctor who is outwardly tense and nervous, either consciously or unconsciously, produces an uncomfortable climate for the doctor–patient encounter.

Clinical students often do not realize that their nervousness and apprehension can impact on the patient's responses in the clinical encounter. It is not unusual for clinical interns to feel somewhat nervous, especially in the beginning, but they should consciously try to develop a confident, relaxed air for the clinical situation. (Clinical students should always remember that a supervising faculty member will always be there to provide guidance and feedback when the student is unsure of how to make a particular decision.)

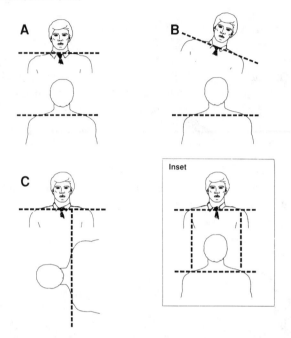

Figure 3.1 Facing the patient squarely. The doctor should face the patient directly, with the axis of the doctor's shoulders parallel to the axis of the patient's shoulders (A). When the doctor faces the patient at a different angle, the doctor may appear uninterested or inattentive (B). At an extreme angle of 90°, the doctor appears to be attending to something totally different from the patient (C). Ideally, the doctor should face the patient directly, as in A. This is referred to as facing the patient *squarely* because imaginary lines connecting the axes of the doctor's and patient's shoulders can be shown to form a square or rectangle (inset).

Muldary (1983) uses the mnemonic CLOSER to describe the six components of good physical attending. A slightly modified explanation of CLOSER, oriented in detail to the doctor–patient interaction, is provided:

C: **CONTROL** distractions and potential interruptions that threaten to interfere with your attention.

L: **LEAN** forward slightly toward the person with whom you are interacting.

O: Maintain an **OPEN**, nondefensive posture, and appear relaxed and at ease in the clinical environment.

S: Face the patient **SQUARELY**, with your shoulders parallel to the patient's.

E: Maintain appropriate **EYE** contact.

R: **RESPECT** the rules of personal space and territoriality.

Table 3.1 Facilitative comments and actions

"Uh-huh"
"Yes"
"Go on"
"and . . ."
"What else?"
"Keep going."
"Tell me more."
"Let's talk more about that."
Head nod "yes"
Reflection
Facilitative, attentive silence

Doctors should listen with their eyes, ears, and body posture. Respecting the rules of space and territoriality is part of making a patient comfortable and at ease in the clinical environment. Further information on personal space and territoriality will be discussed in Chapter 4 (pp. 58–59). With good listening attitudes and physical attending skills, the doctor can become (as Muldary suggests) "CLOSER" to patients.

USE OF FACILITATIVE TECHNIQUES

Facilitative techniques include both verbal and nonverbal cues. Body language is a nonverbal form of facilitation. The listener who leans forward in the chair and uses good eye contact and receptive facial expressions demonstrates active listening.

Several facilitative techniques have been described in Chapter 2 in the context of performing the clinical interview. Any statements or actions that encourage the speaker to continue are facilitative. These include the use of open-ended statements, clarifying statements (reflection, paraphrasing, and summarizing), and validation. Table 3.1 shows a set of words and actions that facilitate further communication. Facilitative, attentive silence is also a nonverbal "encourager" that prompts the patient to continue. By remaining quiet and appearing attentive, the doctor creates a supportive atmosphere for the patient to continue.

Reflection is a particularly useful facilitative technique in which a listener repeats parts of what a speaker says to try to get the speaker to continue:

PATIENT: I keep waking up each morning recently and my eyes are red and itchy.

DOCTOR: Red and itchy?

PATIENT: Yes, they look red and they feel very irritated.

Reflection helps by demonstrating to a speaker that you heard what was just said. This is an active demonstration of good listening that invites the speaker to continue.

EMPATHY

Empathy is the ability to put oneself in another person's position—to feel how another person feels and to experience the other person's perspective. Anderson (1990) describes empathy as "a type of intellectual role playing" in which you attempt to understand the other person's life, problems, values, and meanings as if they were your own.

Covey (1989) presents an example that demonstrates the meaning of empathy. That it involves an optometrist makes the example perfectly suited for a discussion on empathy for eye care professionals:

> Suppose you've been having trouble with your eyes and you decide to go to an optometrist for help. After briefly listening to your complaint, he takes off his glasses and hands them to you.
>
> "Put these on," he says. "I've worn this pair of glasses for ten years now and they've really helped me. I have an extra pair at home; you can wear these."
>
> So you put them on, but it only makes the problem worse.
>
> "This is terrible!" you exclaim. "I can't see a thing!"
>
> "Well what's wrong?" he asks. "They work great for me. Try harder."
>
> "I am trying," you insist. "Everything is a blur."
>
> "Well, what's the matter with you? Think positively."
>
> "Okay. I positively can't see a thing."
>
> "Boy, are you ungrateful!" he chides. "And after all I've done to help you!"

In the case above, the optometrist can see things only from his own viewpoint—through his own eyes. His inability to see things from the other person's viewpoint makes him unable to help his patient.

Empathy is not the same as sympathy. Sympathy is feeling *for* somebody else; it does not necessarily involve sharing the other person's emotions. Sympathy usually involves taking on feelings of sorrow and sadness. In contrast, empathy means feeling *with* another individual; it allows you to capture and understand the other person's feelings, *while maintaining your own identity.*

The objectivity of empathy makes this sentiment a better response for the clinician. As Levinson (1987) points out, "the last thing a distressed patient needs is a distressed caretaker." Anderson (1990) says "Empathy is seeing the world through another person's eyes rather than weeping at the

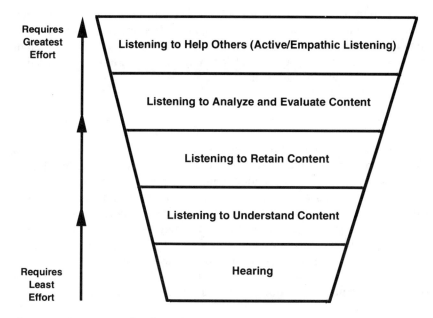

Figure 3.2 Listening level involvement scale. Hearing and listening occur at different levels. Hearing is the lowest level. Empathic listening is the highest level and requires the greatest effort. (Modified from Gamble TK, Gamble MW. Communication Works, 2nd ed. New York: McGraw-Hill, 1987.)

plight of another." With empathy, doctors have the opportunity to share in the feelings of the patient, without the risk of becoming disempowered by these feelings. This is clearly a more therapeutic response.

How can one display empathy?

Listen actively.

Invite patients to share their feelings and concerns.

Use open-ended questions and other facilitative techniques.

Project appropriate nonverbal cues.

Use supportive touch effectively (see Chapter 4, pp. 59–61).

THE LISTENING LEVEL INVOLVEMENT SCALE

Different levels of hearing and listening are demonstrated in the listening level involvement scale (Figure 3.2). Hearing is the lowest of the five levels and requires the least effort. The higher the level of listening, the more energy and effort is required. Listening to *understand* content requires less energy than listening to *retain* content; listening to analyze and evaluate content requires still more energy. Empathic listening, which involves listening to help others, requires the highest level of energy. Good listening is clearly an active process, and listening at the highest level requires personal commitment and effort.

LISTENING STYLES

Examining different listening styles can provide insights into how we listen. A variety of learning styles have been identified in communications (Lunenburg and Ornstein 1991; Freshour 1989). The styles are not mutually exclusive. A listener uses predominantly one type, with a weaker tendency toward one or more of the other styles. In different situations, we may listen differently. During scientific lectures, we may listen primarily with one style; with patients, we may listen predominantly with another.

A set of listening styles, relative to the clinical setting, will be discussed. These include the answer-oriented listener, the technical listener, the stylistic listener, the judgmental listener, and the empathic listener.

The Answer-Oriented Listener

Answer-oriented listeners are listening primarily for the answer to the question that they have asked. If the patient provides other useful information, the doctor may miss these details.

> DOCTOR: Ms. Weathers, do you see things clearly at distance? (The doctor inquires about the patient's distance vision.)
>
> PATIENT: Yes, I see things far away fine. Sometimes when I am reading the newspaper it's a little difficult, but things that are far away are fine. (The doctor records "Distance Vision—no problems" in the patient's record. Having listened for the information looked for, the doctor continues with the rest of the agenda.)
>
> DOCTOR: How about things at near? Do you see well at near? (The doctor missed the patient's comment above about the newspaper. If adequate attention had been paid, the doctor could have continued from the patient's cue about reading, rather than coming across to the patient as inattentive.)

The Technical Listener

The technical listener is very detail-oriented. Preoccupied with details, the doctor may lose sight of the meaning of the full communication. The technical listener often misses cues to a patient's feelings and emotions.

Clinical students often focus on specific details, failing to integrate the whole picture. The technical listener must learn how to handle details and put information together.

The Stylistic Listener

This type of listener is very attentive to the speaker's dress, style, and mannerisms, and often spends more time attending to the *presentation* than to the content of the patient's communication. The stylistic listener is usually very observant of a patient's nonverbal cues and messages. The excessive interest in the nonverbal cues interferes with the doctor's attention to the content and details of the patient's message. This type of listener can benefit by concentrating more on listening to the *content* of the communication, and not letting the "stylistic" factors overshadow the content of the message.

The Judgmental Listener

The judgmental listener is constantly evaluating everything heard and tends to make rapid judgments before a full communication has been given.

This listener often lets personal biases, attitudes, values, and beliefs cloud the clinical situation, and may make unfounded conclusions about a patient based on the patient's background, age, socioeconomic position, educational level, and/or financial status. These clinicians are quick to "label" patients as uncooperative, hostile, or angry, even when the difficulty may be caused by the quality of the doctor–patient interaction. This listener can benefit by remaining more objective, by avoiding premature conclusions, and by concentrating more on the patient's message.

The Empathic Listener

This type of listener is very skilled at understanding the content and feelings of a patient's communications. Doctors with this style are usually very effective in putting the patient at ease in the clinical setting and in getting the patient to cooperate. By remaining attentive to the content and details expressed by the patient, this doctor can get the full meaning of a communication and can be optimally effective. It is this category of listening that provides the deepest and fullest understanding of a message. Empathic listening is a most effective listening style, both inside and outside the clinical setting.

Effective listening helps the doctor obtain more information about the patient. This can improve the doctor's ability in clinical testing, diagnosis, and formation of management plans.

STRATEGIES FOR IMPROVING LISTENING IN THE CLINICAL ENVIRONMENT

1. Develop positive listening attitudes. Become interested in your patients, their stories, and their lives. Much of what they tell you can help you to help them.
2. Listen actively to your patients. Maintain eye contact and use facilitative techniques (e.g., reflection, paraphrasing, summarizing) to show that you are listening.
3. Concentrate on what the patient is saying. Learn to focus your thinking, and do not let your mind wander. Monitor your listening from time to time to make sure that you are still concentrating on the patient. When you are in the examination room with a patient, all that should matter at that moment is the patient. Avoid thoughts of personal matters, financial dilemmas, or office concerns. Do not think about the patient who was in earlier. Do not think about your plans for later that evening. All that should matter for those moments when you are with a patient is that patient.
4. Keep an open mind. Do not make premature conclusions and assumptions and do not let biases and personal values affect your perception of what is said. Listeners who let their own attitudes and beliefs overshadow what is said tend to modify the intended meaning of a message.
5. Listen with your eyes as well as your ears. Good eye contact is a basic way of demonstrating that you are listening. In addition, good body language demonstrates a receptiveness to the speaker. Physically attending and orienting to the patient are essential components of active listening.
6. Listen to verbal *and* nonverbal messages. There is more to communication than words. Nonverbal cues are a valuable part of the communication process.
7. Use good listening skills as one of your techniques for developing good doctor–patient rapport. A doctor's "people skills" are one of the major factors that patients use in evaluating their health care professionals (Leebov et al. 1990). Patients who have good relationships with their doctors report greater levels of satisfaction in the care that they receive.
8. Know how to feel and demonstrate empathy for your patients. Empathy can contribute to your relationships with your patients and to the

quality of care that you provide. Remember that empathic listening is the highest level on the listening level involvement scale.

9. Do not be afraid of silence. Many people get nervous at the prospect of silence, so they start talking. Brief periods of silence in a conversation can contribute to a meaningful interaction between two individuals. Use silence confidently.

10. Above all, to listen you need to face the patient, appear interested, and STOP TALKING!

QUESTIONS FOR THOUGHT

1. How do you demonstrate active listening when you conduct a case history? Do your patients perceive you as an active listener?
2. How can you keep your mind from wandering during the case history?
3. What are common obstacles to listening in the clinical environment? What potential obstacles are present in your environment? How can these be eliminated or reduced?
4. Define empathy. How is empathy different from sympathy? How can you demonstrate empathy to patients?
5. What is meant when we say that it would be "difficult, if not impossible, to provide ethical care without listening to the patient's concerns and desires?" If clinicians are the experts, shouldn't they know what is right for the patient?
6. You are providing some recommendations to a patient at the end of the examination and you get the impression that the patient is not listening to you. You can tell that the patient is tired and is in a rush to leave. The patient came in specifically for new reading glasses, and you are providing a new prescription. But you are concerned that the patient is not listening to you with respect to the increased intraocular pressures. What can you do to encourage the patient to listen to you?
7. Think of a time when you have observed a disagreement or a conflict between two people. Were both individuals listening to each other? Was part of the conflict a result of ineffective communications? How could the two people have communicated more effectively to resolve their disagreement?

REFERENCES

Anderson CA. Patient Teaching and Communicating in an Information Age. Albany, NY: Delmar Publishers, 1990.

Beckman HB, Frankel RM. The effect of physician behavior on the collection of data. Annals of Internal Medicine 101:692–696, 1984.

Covey SR. The Seven Habits of Highly Effective People. New York: Simon & Schuster, 1989.

Freshour FW. Listening power: Key to effective leadership. Illinois School and Research Development 26:17–23, 1989.

Gamble TK, Gamble MW. Communication Works, 2nd ed. New York: McGraw-Hill, 1987.

Korsch BM, Negrete V. Doctor–patient communication. Scientific American 227(August):66–74, 1972.

Levinson D. A Guide to the Clinical Interview. Philadelphia: W.B. Saunders, 1987.

Leebov W, Vergare M, Scott G. Patient Satisfaction: A Guide to Practice Enhancement. Oradell, NJ: Medical Economics Books, 1990.

Lucas SE. The Art of Public Speaking. New York: Random House, 1989.

Lunenberg FC, Ornstein AC. Educational Administration: Concepts and Practices. Belmont, CA: Wadsworth, 1991.

Muldary TW. Interpersonal Relations for Health Professionals. New York: Macmillan, 1983.

Pryor F. The Energetic Manager. Englewood Cliffs, NJ: Prentice Hall, 1987.

ADDITIONAL READINGS

Baker WJ. Listening will improve your hearing. Optometric Management 22:57–61, 1987.

DeVito JA. Human Communication—The Basic Course. New York: Harper & Row, 1988.

DeVito JA. Messages—Building Interpersonal Communication Skills. New York: Harper & Row, 1990.

Mader TF, Mader DC. Understanding One Another—Communicating Interpersonally. Dubuque, IA: William C. Brown, 1990.

Myerscough PR. Talking with Patients—A Basic Clinical Skill. Oxford: Oxford University Press, 1989.

Spiro H. What is empathy and can it be taught? Annals of Internal Medicine 116:843–846, 1992.

Stewart J, D'Angelo G. Together—Communicating Interpersonally. New York: Random House, 1988.

Nonverbal Communication Skills

4

Not all that is communicated is transmitted through words. The nonverbal cues that accompany a verbal message have a significant impact on the way people respond to communication. These cues include body language, personal space and territoriality, use of touch and time, and dress and personal appearance.

In a typical two-person conversation, research indicates that the verbal channel accounts for less than 35% of the way a message is interpreted, and that nonverbal cues account for more than 65% of the meaning (Gamble and Gamble 1987). With less than 35% of the meaning of a message derived directly from the words, good communicators are skilled at attending to, and using, nonverbal signs and cues. Nonverbal communications involve a number of areas including body language, personal space and territoriality, use of touch and time, and dress and physical appearance.

Nonverbal cues can support or contrast with the verbal message and have a significant impact on the interaction between the doctor and patient (Table 4.1). When nonverbal cues correspond with the verbal narrative, the nonverbal cues help to strengthen the delivery of the message. When nonverbal cues do not match the verbal message, it is believed that most people rely more on the nonverbal cues in interpreting the message, and that they pay greater attention to the nonverbal messages (Levinson 1987). Such is the impact and importance of nonverbal communications.

Table 4.1 Cues to nonverbal communications in the clinical environment

Body language (kinesics)
    Gestures
    Body movements
    Facial expressions
    Eye contact
    Posture
Paralanguage
    Intonation
    Rate of speaking
    Pitch
    Volume
    Use of pauses
Space and territoriality (proxemics)
    Horizontal and vertical space
Touch
Time
Physical appearance

In Chapter 1, models of communication showed that communication is a cycle in which the "sender" transmits a message to the "receiver." In *verbal* communications, the speaker (the "sender") also projects nonverbal messages and cues. The active listener is adept at recognizing these non-verbal signs and cues, in addition to attending to the verbal content of the message.

THE IMPACT OF NONVERBAL COMMUNICATIONS

Consider the following two scenarios of a doctor greeting a patient at the beginning of an examination:

A: DOCTOR: Good morning. I'm Dr. Harper. We'll be going down the hall to the room on the right, and I'll be examining you today. My assistant told me that you tore an old contact lens and that you need a new lens right away. She said that you're going to be traveling out of the country. It's a good thing that you came in for the lenses before you left.

B: DOCTOR: Good morning (smiling). I'm Dr. Harper. We'll be going down the hall to the room on the right, and I'll be examining you today (extending arm for a warm handshake). My assistant told me that you tore an old contact lens and that you need a new pair right away. She said that you're going to be traveling out of the country. It's a good thing that you came in for the lenses before you left (friendly tone, smiling).

In scenario A, it is hard to tell whether the doctor is addressing the patient in a warm, courteous tone or a lecturing, pedantic tone. In the second scenario, it is clear that the doctor is speaking in a friendly, caring tone.

BODY LANGUAGE

Facial expressions, body movements, gestures, eye contact, and posture can all have an impact on the way a listener interprets a speaker's message. "Reading" a patient's body language can reveal a lot of information to the doctor. A patient who sits in the examination room tapping her feet on the floor and biting her nails may be perceived as a nervous, anxious patient. A patient with jaws tightly clenched, forehead furrowed, and holding hand to forehead may be evaluated as someone who is in pain. The doctor can learn a lot about the patient by watching the patient's body language. Similarly, the patient learns a lot about the doctor by watching his or her body language.

The components that comprise body language, or kinesics (e.g., gestures, body movements, facial expressions, eye contact, and posture) range across a wide spectrum. During normal conversation, facial expressions are a significant part of the communication process, especially since the listener is already looking at the speaker's face. Making eye contact with a person is one of the fastest ways to initiate a conversation and to establish a bond of communication with the individual. Lack of eye contact during the conversation may be perceived as a sign that the communicator is distracted, bored, uninterested, dishonest, embarrassed, or shy. During a case history, the patient who does not receive eye contact from the doctor may think that the doctor is thinking about something else, or that the doctor does not care. Direct and steady eye contact makes a speaker appear confident, firm, and steadfast. For the listener, maintaining eye contact is a way of demonstrating one's attention to the other individual.

The doctor's body posture and language can convey important messages about the doctor's self-confidence and self-esteem. The way doctors feel about and carry themselves will affect how patients feel about the doctor. In addition, posture and body language can indicate the doctor's receptiveness to the patient. An open body position, with a forward lean to the body, is seen as an attentive body posture (see Chapter 3).

Nonverbal indicators projected by the doctor may also suggest a "friendly" or "unfriendly" climate to the patient. A warm "hello" with an accompanying smile, handshake, and eye contact may make a patient feel comfortable and welcome to the doctor's office.

SYNCHRONY AND PACING

Synchrony refers to the degree of harmony between the nonverbal behaviors of the doctor and patient. Matching or pacing a patient's nonverbal behaviors can build rapport and empathy (Cormier and Cormier 1991). If the patient is leaning forward, with hands crossed over the lap, the doctor should assume a similar body posture. If the patient displays a facial expression of frustration or confusion while speaking, the doctor should demonstrate a congruent expression. Pacing refers to moving as the patient moves. These actions must be done subtly to be effective.

PARALANGUAGE

Paralanguage consists of vocal cues such as intonation, rate of speaking, pitch, and volume. These cues contribute to the meaning of the message and have the ability to change the meaning of a verbal communication. The use of pauses during communication is also an important element of paralanguage.

INTONATION

Intonation has been called "the melody of speech" (Anderson 1990). This component of communications provides emphasis on words that affects the interpreted meaning of the message. Consider how the different intonations indicated in the sentences below change the interpretation and meaning of the message; notice that the words are identical, but changes in intonation change the meaning:

I will *not* clean my contact lenses nightly.

I will not clean my contact lenses *nightly*.

I will not clean my contact lenses nightly.

In the first sentence, the speaker seems most concerned about the cleaning process, in the second the speaker seems more concerned about the cleaning schedule having to be done *nightly*, and in the third the speaker seems most concerned about who is to do the cleaning. The words in the sentences are identical, but different intonation produces different meanings.

RATE OF SPEECH

Since different people process information at different rates, doctors may want to adjust their rate for a particular patient. Older patients who have experienced some hearing deficits may prefer slower rates of speaking to give them time to process what they have heard and to clarify any uncertainties. When communicating with a patient who primarily speaks a foreign language, the doctor may find that a slower rate may give the patient more time to interpret and process the information.

PITCH

Pitch refers to tone—the highness or lowness—of the speaker's voice. Women tend to speak in higher pitches than men. Hearing deficits associated with aging tend to be higher pitch (higher frequency) deficits, so a lower pitch may be more easily understood by an elderly patient with a hearing problem (Anderson 1990).

VOLUME

Volume refers to the loud or quiet nature of the speaker's voice. Vibrant speakers tend to alternate the loudness and softness of their phrases. Changing one's volume can be a helpful tool in the clinic. Changing one's volume can be used to reenergize a patient, adult or child, who appears to be fatiguing during an examination.

USE OF PAUSES

Skillful speakers use brief pauses and silence in communications. Although we generally concentrate on *what is said* when we think of communications, the use of silence is a valuable factor in successful speaking. Many people feel nervous at the thought of "quiet" space in conversation, but pauses can allow listeners to reflect on what has been heard, and to think about what they want to say next. Many people who are uncomfortable with the brief silent interludes in conversation tend to substitute distractors (e.g., um's, ehr's, and uh's) in place of the silence; this may give them time to think, but it does little to contribute to the quality of the communication, and it may distract the listener who is trying to make sense of what is said.

When used correctly, silence should be considered an asset to communications. The clinician should feel comfortable with using brief pauses and silence. Patients may appreciate the time in which they can process the

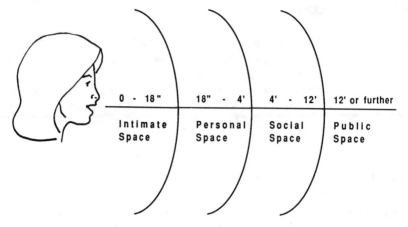

Figure 4.1 Categories of space in proxemics. Four types of distances are illustrated: intimate space, personal space, social space, and public space. When an individual's personal and intimate space are invaded, the individual may feel uncomfortable or apprehensive.

information, and pauses may provide a more relaxed element to the doctor–patient interaction.

SPACE AND PROXEMICS

Proxemics, or space and territoriality, is an important part of interpersonal communications. We have frequently heard the warning "not to invade someone's personal space." A person's physical territory and personal space are intimately tied to his or her feeling of identity and individuality. Respecting personal space is an unspoken rule in good communications.

Four different distances are described in Figure 4.1. During normal interpersonal communications, we are generally at a personal distance from our communication partner. Coming closer than that can sometimes make the partner anxious or uncomfortable. In the clinical environment, we are generally at a personal distance, too; however, in the clinical setting there are times, such as when performing ophthalmoscopy, when the doctor has to go within what is considered a person's intimate distance. The doctor should be aware that this may result in feelings of discomfort and apprehension in some patients.

How can the doctor make the patient more comfortable when invading the patient's intimate space during a procedure? Informing the patient just before starting a procedure that it is necessary to come close to examine the patient's eyes can help to prepare the patient. Explaining the significance of the procedure can also help to justify why the close range is necessary. Patients usually understand that doctors have to do some procedures at a close distance, but providing a sensitive explanation, and warning in advance, can help make the patient more comfortable.

Special dimensions of proxemics involve the use of horizontal and vertical space. The variations of horizontal space, the nearness or distance between communicators, has been discussed. Vertical space, the up-and-down distance between patients, is also important in communicating. It is preferable for both the doctor and the patient to be at the same height (Figure 4.2). A setting in which the doctor is positioned higher or lower than the patient perpetuates the message that the doctor and patient are not "equals." A setting in which the doctor is seated much higher than the patient may be seen as perpetuating the image of the doctor being "more important" than the patient. Further, when the two are not at eye level, there may be physical discomfort in one or both of the individuals, in bending the neck to look up (or down) at each other. Communicators who face each other at eye level are more likely seen as equals in the interaction. Comfortable, equal communication occurs with the doctor and patient at eye level, at about the same vertical height.

TOUCH

Touch tests the nearest limits of territoriality, because it involves actual physical contact between individuals. Touch can also be one of the most direct and intense forms of communication. A supportive touch to the shoulder of the patient who appears nervous and anxious may help to soothe and calm the person.

Like eye contact, touch can be a very powerful means of forming a communication bond. Touch, however, is a sensitive, emotional issue because of misinterpretations that can take place. Clinicians usually use touch as a sign of caring and understanding and reassurance and support; touch can also be interpreted as a sign of affection and a physical interest in the other individual.

It is important for doctors to be sure that their touch is interpreted in the way it was intended. Being sensitive to a patient's response when he or she is touched can help the doctor perceive how the touch is accepted. Nonverbal cues are very helpful in sensing how another individual is responding to touch. Some patients may respond favorably, perhaps looking more relaxed and at ease, and some may appear to tense up and take on a more stiff, rigid posture. The doctor who sees that a patient is not responding well to touch should withdraw the hand, sensing that this patient does not appreciate the physical contact. Some

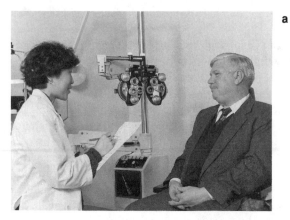

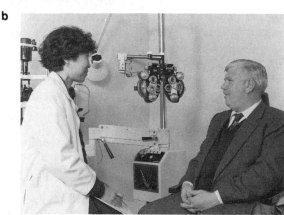

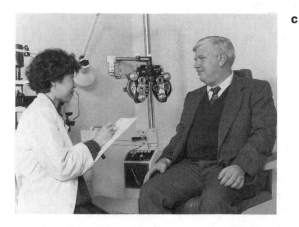

Figure 4.2 Sitting at the same vertical height. The doctor and patient should be seated at eye level (a). An arrangement in which the doctor is positioned higher (b) or lower (c) than the patient perpetuates the image that doctors and patients are "unequals."

patients do not like to be touched, even if the intent is one of caring and support.

With older patients, nervous patients, and children, using touch appropriately can be a particularly valuable tool in conveying a sense of caring and concern to the patient. The doctor must bear in mind that some patients will appreciate this form of communication and some will not. If used appropriately, however, the power of touch can be a valuable asset in the doctor's ability to communicate and reach patients.

A handshake at the beginning of the examination, as the doctor greets the patient, is an example of touch that occurs initially in the doctor–patient encounter, and is a way that the doctor has of "reaching out" to the patient. The handshake is a "socially acceptable" application of "touch"; thus, it is not threatening or open to misinterpretation as other forms of touch may be. The handshake at the start of the examination is helpful in forming the initial linkage between the doctor and patient. Touch during the rest of the examination can also be very useful in building doctor–patient rapport and in communicating with patients.

TIME

Do patients feel rushed by a clinician? Although time is not often thought of as a factor of communication, the doctor's use of time can send important messages to the patient. Providing patients with appropriate time for their examinations is one of the doctor's ways of saying "I care" about the patient. In addition, a patient who does not feel time-pressured may be more relaxed and at ease, and the level of patient cooperation may be greater during the examination. Thus, time can affect the quality of the doctor–patient interaction, and it can also affect the quality of care that the patient receives.

Doctors who consistently run behind in their offices and keep patients waiting are sometimes perceived as disrespectful of the patient's time. Although it is sometimes unavoidable to be behind in one's schedule, maintaining a sense of time in the office is imperative.

When the doctor is running behind, it is a sign of courtesy if the doctor or an assistant explains to the waiting patients that there is an unavoidable delay, and that the doctor will be with them as soon as possible. Patients usually understand occasional delays, if they do not occur consistently. Additional time needed with some patients (e.g., hearing impaired, elderly patients, anxious patients, foreign language patients) can improve the doctor–patient encounter and should be scheduled accordingly. A factor in communication, time plays a role in the way a doctor interacts with the patient.

DRESS AND PERSONAL APPEARANCE

Personal appearance can play a role in a patient's perception of the doctor's confidence and self-esteem. By appearing professional and neat, the doctor projects an image of respect and dignity. Personal appearance also plays a part in first impressions. Dressing appropriately is a way of communicating that "you are important to me." If the doctor comes to the office untidy and disheveled, then a patient may perceive this as a sign that the doctor did not consider the clinical encounter important enough to dress appropriately.

A doctor's observation of personal appearance in a patient is also a factor of communication. A patient whose physical appearance has recently become haggard and pale may reflect the physical manifestations of an illness. The elderly patient who suddenly begins to show poor personal hygiene and grooming may be demonstrating his or her difficulty in carrying out various cleaning and grooming activities. A patient's self-esteem and emotional state may also be reflected in changes in personal hygiene and appearance. Depressed patients, for example, and those with lowered self-esteem may start to dress poorly, and may cease caring for themselves appropriately. The astute clinician who recognizes these cues can be helpful in identifying various problems that result from illness.

The physical appearance of both the doctor and the patient are important factors in communication, and can play a role in the doctor–patient interaction.

STRATEGIES FOR IMPROVING NONVERBAL COMMUNICATIONS IN THE CLINICAL ENVIRONMENT

1. Remember that researchers have found that doctors who are more sensitive to nonverbal communications, such as body posture and space, attain greater levels of patient satisfaction (Cohen-Cole 1991). Consider how your nonverbal communications impact on your interactions with patients.
2. Become more attuned to the way in which body language, paralanguage, and physical space contribute to your communications. By making appropriate use of these components, a doctor can convey a caring and supportive attitude.
3. Mirroring and pacing can be valuable assets in demonstrating empathy and building rapport. Remember that to be effective, synchrony must be displayed in a natural, unpresuming manner.

4. Understand the four different levels of horizontal distance (intimate distance, personal distance, social distance, and public distance). When you must perform a clinical examination that requires you to come very close to the patient, let the patient know in advance that you will be approaching.
5. In addition to horizontal distance, effective use of vertical distance can affect the interaction between the doctor and patient.
6. Judicious use of touch can also be a powerful way to "reach out" to patients. However, remember that not all patients appreciate being touched.
7. Physical appearance and time management in the clinical environment also affect communications.

QUESTIONS FOR THOUGHT

1. What impact do your nonverbal communication skills have in the way your patients respond to you?
2. It is believed that when nonverbal cues conflict with the verbal message, people rely more on nonverbal cues in interpreting the message. Why is this so?
3. Play a 10-minute part of a videotape (e.g., movie, television show) that includes an interpersonal conversation between two people. *Only listen* to the tape, do not watch it. At the end of 10 minutes, think about all you know about each of the people, the environment, and the situation. Now, play the tape again, but this time watch *and* listen to the tape. What additional information did you elicit from the tape this time? What conclusions can you make about the importance of nonverbal cues to communications?
4. Have yourself videotaped while performing an examination, or watch a colleague conduct an examination. As you observe, watch the doctor's nonverbal communications throughout the examination. How do facial expressions, posture, eye contact, and gestures affect the communications? How does the doctor use paralanguage (e.g., vocal intonation, speed of speaking, pitch, volume, and use of pauses)?
5. Work with a partner, and take turns "mirroring" each other's gestures and nonverbal behaviors. Each partner should practice synchrony and pacing for a 10-minute period. Try to make your actions appear natural, unaccentuated movements that resemble mimicking.
6. How are the concepts of personal space and territoriality involved in the clinical environment? When you need to come close to the patient, as in ophthalmoscopy, what can you do to make the experience more comfortable for the patient?

7. What role does the sense of touch play in the delivery of clinical care? Under what conditions can it be helpful to touch a patient? When would you want to avoid touching a patient?
8. How does a doctor's appearance affect a patient's impression of the doctor?

REFERENCES

Anderson CA. Patient Teaching and Communicating in an Information Age. Albany, NY: Delmar Publishers, 1990.

Cohen-Cole SA. The Medical Interview: The Three-Function Approach. St. Louis, MO: Mosby Year Book, 1991.

Cormier WH, Cormier LS. Interviewing Strategies for Helpers. Pacific Grove, CA: Brooks/Cole, 1991.

Gamble TK, Gamble MW. Communication Works, 2nd ed. New York: McGraw-Hill, 1987.

Levinson DL. A Guide to the Clinical Interview. Philadelphia: W.B. Saunders, 1987.

ADDITIONAL READINGS

Axtell RE. Gestures—The Do's and Taboos of Body Language Around the World. New York: John Wiley, 1991.

DeVito JA. Human Communication—The Basic Course. New York: Harper & Row, 1988.

DeVito JA. Messages—Building Interpersonal Communication Skills. New York: Harper & Row, 1990.

Lucas SE. The Art of Public Speaking. New York: Random House, 1989.

Mader TF, Mader DC. Understanding One Another—Communicating Interpersonally. Dubuque IA: William C. Brown, 1990.

Okun FB. Effective Helping Interviewing and Counseling Techniques. Pacific Grove, CA: Brooks/Cole, 1992.

Pearson JC, Nelson PE. Understanding and Sharing—An Introduction to Speech Communication. Dubuque, IA: William C. Brown, 1988.

Stewart J, D'Angelo G. Together—Communicating Interpersonally. New York: Random House, 1988.

5

Delivering Bad News: Supportive Communication

As doctors, our goals are traditionally to cure, heal, and solve problems. Unfortunately, there are times when these objectives are not possible and it becomes necessary to deliver bad news.

The doctor's delivery can make a significant difference in how the patient receives bad news. By monitoring the patient's responses during the conversation, the doctor can obtain cues about how to proceed with additional information (Cohen-Cole 1991; Anderson 1990; Alpert and Wittenberg 1986). By addressing the topic with empathy, sensitivity, honesty, and compassion, the doctor can help the patient deal realistically and practically with the news that must be shared.

When discussing vision loss with patients, eye doctors should be familiar with the types of concerns that patients have. These may include fear of diminished independence, fear of "going blind," fear of decreased function and abilities, fear of embarrassment in front of friends and colleagues, and fear of losing control of one's body and self. These feelings are often accompanied by a changing self-image, especially if patients perceive that their impairment will interfere with their job status, family relationships, reputation, or power. When a patient has a serious medical problem, there is generally a period of mourning in which the patient learns to adjust to the loss. The actual sequence and intensity of emotions are believed to be quite variable from one patient to another. Discussing vision loss with patients is challenging (Klein and Klein 1987; Herrin 1983), but the doctor who is familiar with the types of emotional responses that occur can be better prepared for these situations (Table 5.1).

DELIVERING THE MESSAGE

When bad news must be transmitted, there are steps that the doctor can take to make the delivery more supportive and effective. A five-step model is presented in Table 5-2.

Preparing the patient to receive the news is an important part of the interaction. This step is often overlooked, but it can make a big difference in how a patient responds to the information. Make sure the patient is comfortable and attentive before starting the discussion. A brief introductory statement can help prepare the patient to receive the news. ("Ms. Connor, I found something during my examination that I would like to discuss with you. I would like to explain what I found, and then we can discuss what we can do about it.") Reminding the patient of presenting symptoms that relate to the diagnosis can also serve as an effective introduction.

When presenting the diagnosis, avoid unnecessary technical language and jargon. Explain any clinical terms in language tailored to the patient's understanding. Consider the patient's goals in determining optimal management plans.

Table 5.1 Emotional responses to bad news

Series of stages according to Kübler-Ross (1969)
    Shock and denial
    Anger
    Bargaining
    Depression
    Acceptance
Major types of psychological reactions according to Blum (1960)
    Depression and self-rejection
    Fear
    Counterphobia
    Anxiety
    Frustration and anger
    Withdrawal or apathy
    Exaggeration of symptoms
    Regression
    Dependency
    Self-centeredness

Table 5.2 Five-step plan for delivering bad news

Prepare the patient

Assess the patient's readiness to listen

Use an introductory statement to prepare the patient for information (e.g., remind patient of presenting symptoms and correlate diagnosis to symptoms)

Make sure the environment is comfortable for the patient

Avoid distractions and make sure that there will be adequate time for discussion

Deliver the message

Be clear, concise, and direct

Avoid "information overload"

When using clinical terms, explain them in simple, understandable terms

"Know your audience" and cater your delivery accordingly (e.g., speed of transmission, use of language, use and interpretation of nonverbal cues)

Give the patient time to process the information

Encourage the patient to ask questions and discuss concerns

Discuss the management plan

Present proposed treatment recommendations and plans

Educate the patient about the full range treatment alternatives, with advantages and disadvantages

Consider the patient's views and priorities in determining optimal management strategies

Express hope for a favorable outcome when appropriate

If prognosis is poor, discuss steps to life style adjustments

Consider how the condition and treatment will impact on the patient's life and ability to function

Review management plans discussed and encourage the patient's commitment and compliance

Monitor the patient's understanding and acceptance

Use feedback to evaluate the patient's response

Invite the patient to call with any concerns or questions

Consider setting up a meeting to discuss follow-up questions

Listen to the patient along both cognitive and affective domains

Facilitate access to support systems

Encourage the patient's access to support systems: relatives, friends, neighbors

Provide information about community resources, support groups, local agencies

Additional tests that are required to confirm a diagnosis or evaluate a patient's status should be explained clearly to the patient. Proposed treatments and therapies must also be discussed in detail. According to the doctrine of informed consent, patients are entitled to know the advantages, risks, and side effects of proposed treatments and alternative forms of therapy that exist. They must also be told the probability for success and the anticipated prognosis in the absence of treatment.

Monitor the patient's understanding of diagnosis and management plans and encourage the patient to discuss questions or concerns. When bad news about children must be delivered, the emotional responses of parents should be considered (Chapter 16). In these situations, the doctor must monitor the responses of both the patient and the parent to assist in the adjustment process (see Case 5.1). When caring for adults, doctors can ask patients for permission to involve relatives and caretakers in discussions about diagnosis and management.

Some doctors try to protect patients from bad news by avoiding difficult issues, but patients are entitled to details about their health status and clinical care. Although it is not possible to modify the bad news, there are certain aspects of delivery that may make the experience easier for the patient. The doctor can control the speed at which information is delivered, the words used to convey the message, and the support accompanying the message. An effective clinician adjusts the combination of these factors to match the patient's level of understanding and need.

CASES INVOLVING UNCERTAINTY

Discussing clinical problems under conditions of uncertainty is a complex task. Sometimes patients are referred for tests to confirm or rule out a potential diagnosis. The underlying question is, should you tell the patient of your working diagnosis? Would telling the patient about the possibility of a serious problem create undue concern, particularly if the patient ends up *not* having the disease? Patients have a right to information that can help them make informed decisions. Arguments for and against providing information in situations that involve uncertainty have been postulated. An open exchange of information gives patients the greatest opportunity to plan for the future and consider their options (Cases 5.2 and 5.3).

HANDLING SITUATIONS WHEN PATIENTS CRY

When patients are forced to come to terms with the diagnosis of serious illnesses (cancer, heart disease, or advanced vision loss), they sometimes start to cry. Crying is a strong emotional response, and it often elicits negative responses from health care professionals. Many doctors are seized with fear when patients even look like they are going to cry. Common responses are to ignore the patient's crying, or to change the subject and talk more, hoping that the patient will automatically turn off the tears. Neither of these actions is facilitative or therapeutic.

It is also sometimes tempting to reassure the patient that "everything is going to be all right" but it is unfair to offer this sentiment unless it is genuine. Sometimes the best a doctor can do is to offer support and show concern.

When patients do begin to cry, the best action is to allow them to express their emotions in a way that they feel is appropriate. This shows that the doctor accepts the patient's emotions and is not trying to interfere with his or her emotional expression. The doctor may wish to offer the patient a tissue, or to offer some words of support. Patients who start to cry may appreciate slightly less direct and less steady eye contact. Some clinicians find it helpful to take a few moments to write in the patient's record to give a patient a few moments in which to become composed. An attitude of support and concern is also comforting.

Patients with glaucoma, macular degeneration, and retinal detachments have realistic concerns. Trying to stop their tears can prevent them from facing their concerns (Cases 5.4 and 5.5). Working to envision the situation from the patient's viewpoint can help a doctor understand what the patient is feeling. The doctor should not suggest problems but should encourage patients to discuss their fears and concerns. Considering possible solutions and alternatives with patients and educating them about available resources can eliminate some of the worries. In some cases, learning to recognize a patient's more subtle cues can help the doctor handle these situations before they escalate to crying. Offering support and giving the patient the freedom to cry are sometimes the most therapeutic actions that can be taken. When handled well, crying can help a patient work toward acceptance. The caring, sensitive doctor can serve a valuable role in these situations.

STRATEGIES FOR DELIVERING BAD NEWS

Delivering bad news is an inescapable function for doctors. There are times when science and technology do not provide the doctor with answers to a patient's problems. When faced with a situation in which bad news must be shared, the doctor should remember the steps that can make the experience more positive for both the doctor and patient.

1. Prepare patients to receive the news, so they are ready to receive the information that will follow. Usually a simple statement such as the following can help brace and prepare the patient for the ensuing discussion: "Mr. Martinez, I would like to discuss some of my findings with you, and explain why you have been having trouble seeing recently."
2. Be direct and concise in delivering the message. Patients are entitled to know when a problem exists. A simple explanation is usually easiest in conveying the information.

3. Do not "overload" the patient with too much information at once. Monitor the patient's understanding of information, control the speed at which information is presented, and choose appropriate words to convey the information. Give the patient an opportunity to ask questions, and listen to assess the patient's level of understanding.
4. Monitor the patient's responses along both the cognitive and affective dimensions. Addressing a patient's comprehension of facts without attending to the patient's emotional status can leave a patient apprehensive. Acceptance involves both a cognitive understanding and an emotional adjustment.
5. Once the bad news has been delivered, present a management plan as soon as possible, so the patient understands what can be done to address the problem.
6. Relatives and caretakers often play a significant role in a patient's compliance and adjustment. With the patient's permission, include them in discussions and encourage their help to ease the patient's adjustment to important life style and functional changes.
7. Be sure that the patient has access to support systems. Inform patients of local agencies and community resources. Patients are usually appreciative when doctors make them aware of these valuable services.
8. Learn to handle situations when patients cry. By handling these encounters effectively, doctors can encourage patients to express their feelings and work toward acceptance.

Case 5.1

Robert is a 16-year-old male. He complains of poor night vision, with no other symptoms. Robert's mother, Ms. Tarrington, says that her older brother also had night vision problems, but that he was killed in an automobile accident at the age of 24, and they never had a diagnosis for his problem.

The doctor finds that Robert's best corrected visual acuities are 20/20 in each eye, at distance and near. During a dilated fundus examination, the doctor finds arteriolar attenuation and bone spicule pigmentation that are typical of retinitis pigmentosa (RP). Visual field defects in the periphery and markedly reduced electrogram findings confirm the diagnosis of RP. The patient and his mother are both concerned. Both are probably wondering about a number of issues, including the deepest fear: is the patient going to go blind? When one child is diagnosed with a problem, parents are often also concerned about whether other children will be affected. Encouraging the patient and family members to ask questions and express their concerns can help the doctor monitor the patient's understanding and acceptance of the diagnosis.

DR. VALLEE: Robert, you talked about the problems that you have seeing at night, and I found some information that helps me understand what is causing your problems. (The doctor looks back and forth between Robert and his mother, to maintain a rapport with both.) You have what is called "retinitis pigmentosa." This is an eye problem in which patients frequently have problems with their night vision. Some people refer to it as "RP." Have you ever heard of RP before? (Give the patient and his mother some time to digest the news.)

MS. TARRINGTON: What else besides night vision is affected? (She demonstrates that she is ready for more information.)

DR. VALLEE: Many people also feel that their side vision is affected. In Robert's case, I am finding only a small decrease in his side vision. Robert, one of the things that I would like to have you do is come back regularly so we can monitor your side vision. (The doctor is beginning to discuss the management plan.)

ROBERT: Is it going to get bad? Am I going to have to wear thick glasses? (Robert is asking the intense question: how bad is it going to get?)

DR. VALLEE: The changes vary in different patients. In some people, the signs remain stable for a long time, and in others they change at a faster pace. (The information is conveyed in a neutral tone, to avoid creating excess worry and concern.) What I would like to do is to see you frequently so we can monitor your progress. You have a very mild prescription now, and the types of changes that occur are not usually the types that are addressed by thick glasses. I will keep you up to date so you will know how you are doing. (The doctor assures the patient and his mother that he will be there for them, and that follow-up is indicated.)

MS. TARRINGTON: What about his younger brothers? Robert has two younger brothers. Do they have it, too?

The doctor continues to respond to the questions of Robert and his mother in a supportive manner. During the discussion of the diagnosis, the doctor listens to the patient's (and caretaker's) lead in determining what additional information is desired. By developing a therapeutic relationship, the doctor improves patient understanding and continuity of care.

Case 5.2

Ms. Arken is a 58-year-old female who works as a driver at a taxi service. She has no personal or family history of glaucoma or ocular disease. Based on the following data obtained from a routine eye examination, does this patient have glaucoma?

Best corrected VAs:
Distance	OD	20/20
	OS	20/20
Near	OD	20/20
	OS	20/20

Ophthalmoscopy
c/d: OD 0.65
           OS 0.70
Disc borders distinct, healthy color
Deep cupping OU
a/v: OD 2/3
       OS 2/3
Macula: Foveal reflex—present OU
Tonometry (applanation):   OD 23, 22
                               OS 23, 22

The doctor determines that the large c/d ratios and borderline intraocular pressures warrant further investigation to rule out the possibility of glaucoma. The doctor asks the patient to return the next morning for visual fields, gonioscopy, and a pressure recheck. How should the doctor explain the results to the patient?

DR. JONTER: Ms. Arken, I have completed the testing for today, but I would like to have you back for some additional tests. Let me tell you why I am making this recommendation.

MS. ARKEN: All right, go on.

DR. JONTER: When I measured the pressures inside your eyes the numbers were in the borderline area—not *terribly* high, but a little above what we usually find. I also found that a measurement in the back of your eyes, on your optic nerves, was large. These are *sometimes*—not always, but sometimes—associated with glaucoma.

MS. ARKEN: Oh, that doesn't sound good.

DR. JONTER: Well, again, Ms. Arken, as I said they are *sometimes* associated. In many cases, patients with these findings do *not* have glaucoma. The only way to find out for sure is to do some further testing. That's why I'd like to have you back for some additional tests. (The doctor continues with a brief explanation of each of the tests, and then answers some questions.)

Case 5.3

Ms. Byler is a 37-year-old female. She has experienced an isolated episode of optic neuritis that has resolved without complication. The etiology is not certain. The doctor is aware that in some cases, optic neuritis is associated with multiple sclerosis. In this case, should the doctor tell the patient about the possibility that she may develop multiple sclerosis?

Slamovits and colleagues (1991) argue that if optic neuritis were associated with multiple sclerosis in 100% of cases, the decision in favor of telling would be easier. Similarly, if the association was remote and very rare, the decision *not* to tell would possibly be a stronger option. Previous studies showed the association to be as low as 11%, but recent studies suggest that it may be closer to 75%. Since the actual association is not established, the decision is still complicated.

Various arguments for and against telling the patient can be made.

1. Yes, the patient should be told of the association.
   a. Patients have a right to details about their health; this information is essential in allowing them to make their life plans.
   b. Since we live in a highly mobile society, and there is no guarantee that a patient will return to you in the future, the doctor should not withhold currently held information.
   c. Information about the association between optic neuritis and multiple sclerosis is frequently cited in the public media and lay publications. It is better for patients to find out about it from the doctor than to read or hear about it themselves.
   d. If patients know they are at risk for a clinical disease, they may make more informed decisions about future medical care and coverage. Waiting until a condition becomes active may put the patient at a disadvantage in seeking medical insurance and disability coverage.
   e. So that she may make more informed decisions about becoming pregnant, a woman of child-bearing age should be made aware of the increased risk of manifestation of multiple sclerosis symptoms as a result of pregnancy.
2. No, why worry the patient needlessly?
   a. The treatment of patients with isolated optic neuritis is not any different from the treatment of optic neuritis related to multiple sclerosis. There are no medical advantages in telling the patient of this potential relationship.
   b. "Labeling" patients with a disease entity that they may not have may cause unnecessary harm and concern.

Discussion:

According to the law of informed consent, patients are entitled to know *unless* the doctor feels that the patient does not want to know, or if the information would be harmful to the patient.

An open exchange of information gives patients the greatest opportunity to consider their options and plan for the future. When receiving bad news, patients are often "paralyzed" with fear and shock, and are unable for a brief time to make decisions. Providing patients with information *in advance* can give them an extended period of time to deal with their feelings and consider their options.

By stressing that the association is not certain, the doctor can help reduce excessive levels of stress and anxiety on the part of the patient. Neither option may appear an overwhelming choice because of the possibility of the alternate outcome. The option of an open, honest disclosure, however, provides the patient with the greatest opportunity to plan and make informed decisions.

Case 5.4

Mr. Parkson is a 68-year-old retired high school English teacher. He has experienced blurred vision of increasing severity over the past year. He presents to the eye doctor hoping to get new glasses to improve his vision. The doctor diagnoses age-related macular degeneration and explains to the patient that this condition is irreversible, but that steps can be taken to minimize additional changes in the future. The doctor observes that Mr. Parkson is distressed by this news, and that he is starting to cry.

DR. KILEY: Mr. Parkson, I can tell that this is very upsetting to you. I can imagine that this must be very disturbing. (The doctor pauses to give the patient a chance to respond and express his concern, and continues when he does not answer.) There is nothing wrong with crying. Sometimes it's the most natural response to a difficult situation.

MR. PARKSON: It's just such a shock. I can't believe that this is what it's going to be like from now on. I used to enjoy reading so much. Now it's a chore.

DR. KILEY: I can understand that reading has become more difficult for you. As I mentioned earlier, there are some special lenses and magnifiers that you may find helpful. Maybe you can think about some of the options that we talked about, and we can meet again so we can discuss them further. (The doctor has briefly discussed the possibility of low vision aids with the patient, but can tell that he is not ready to handle further information at this time. The doctor feels that he may be more receptive in the future, and encourages him to return when he is ready. By encouraging him to return, long-term concern and support for him are expressed. By allowing him to express his emotions and fears, the doctor is seen by the patient as a caring and concerned practitioner. He will probably be comfortable returning to the doctor's care in the future.)

Case 5.5

Ms. Westerman is a 52-year-old female who has had recent complaints of blurred vision and floaters. The doctor has identified that there is a retinal detachment. As the doctor explains this to the patient and describes that she will need retinal surgery, the patient starts to cry.

DR. BLOOM: I can tell that this is upsetting, Ms. Westerman. I am sure that you weren't expecting this.

MS. WESTERMAN: No, not at all. Things can be going along fine, and all of a sudden something like this occurs.

DR. BLOOM: Yes, it can be very difficult, especially when it is unexpected. (The doctor shows empathy for the patient's concerns.) The good thing is that there is something that we can do about this to maintain your vision.

(The doctor gives the patient a little time to process the information and organize her thoughts, and then continues when she appears ready for additional information.) Ms. Westerman, let's talk a little bit more about what we can do to help you. I would be happy to refer you to an excellent retinal surgeon. I have worked with this surgeon for a very long time, and know that this person does an excellent job. (In this case, the patient does not have time to think about the options and return to discuss them later, as in the previous case. Retinal surgery must be performed right away. By instilling confidence in the surgeon, Dr. Bloom can make the patient feel more secure about the procedure that must be done. When the patient is ready for more information, the doctor explains exactly what the procedure encompasses. The doctor calls the surgeon to initiate the referral, sets up the appointment for the patient, offers to answer any questions, and then reminds the patient that she will be seen again following the surgery. By providing reassurance to the patient and encouraging her to express her concerns and questions, the doctor helps the patient through a difficult experience.)

QUESTIONS FOR THOUGHT

1. A 49-year-old female was examined in a comprehensive eye examination. Her chief concerns were the occurrence of headaches and blurred vision at near. The headaches used to occur about once a month, but now she says that they are occurring more frequently. She feels that she must need new glasses to eliminate the headaches. You find that she needs new glasses for reading, but you also perform a visual field examination because of her history of headaches. You find that she has a bitemporal hemianopia and you are considering the possibility of a pituitary tumor. You are going to refer this patient for a CT scan and to a neurologist for further care. How do you discuss this news with the patient?

2. A 32-year-old male presents for a general eye examination with no symptoms or visual complaints. During ophthalmoscopy, you see cotton wool spots on both retinas. He says that he had a complete physical examination two months ago, and you can rule out most problems such as diabetes and hypertension. You are considering the possibility of HIV infection. How do you bring this topic up with the patient? What do you say, and how do you discuss this concern?

3. Consider the following two cases:
   a. You examine a 62-year-old patient who has presented for a routine eye examination with no symptoms. You find a peripheral retinal detachment.
   b. You examine a 62-year-old patient who has presented with symptoms of light flashes and floaters. You find a retinal detachment extending from the mid-periphery, temporal to the macula.

Both patients have a retinal detachment. One has symptoms, and the other does not. Is there any difference in your explanation to these two patients?

4. You examine a 69-year-old female and find that she has had irreversible vision loss. The patient has limited visual fields in both eyes resulting from uncontrolled glaucoma. She was diagnosed five years ago by another doctor, but did not go to that doctor regularly because "my eye didn't hurt, and my vision wasn't blurry." Now she is aware of significant constrictions in her visual field and she has come to you in search of a solution to her current vision problems. How do you discuss this with the patient?

5. A 57-year-old male had an episode of fluctuating diplopia and ptosis; the symptoms disappeared after a brief period of time. He returns to your office 18 months later, indicating that the symptoms have returned. The diplopia varies during the day, getting worse at the end of the day. The ptosis also varies. You are considering a possible diagnosis of myasthenia gravis. You want to schedule the patient for a Tensilon (edrophonium chloride) test. Should you inform the patient of your working diagnosis?

6. A mother and father accompany their 5-year-old daughter for an eye examination. They think that she may need glasses, and observe that she sometimes has trouble seeing. You examine her and find that she has congenital toxoplasmosis, with a large area of the macula affected. How do you discuss this with the parents and the child?

7. A 7-year-old male is brought in for an eye examination. He has no problems seeing clearly at distance and near, and his parents tell you that he is doing very well in school. They mention that he has always had problems identifying colors, but aside from that they have no concerns. You perform a color vision test and find that he has a color vision defect of protanopia. How do you discuss this finding?

8. A 76-year-old female has dense cataracts, and she has a presurgical work-up to determine the potential benefits of cataract surgery. It is determined that she has extensive retinal scarring in both eyes resulting from long-standing diabetic retinopathy, with an old retinal detachment in the right eye. The optometrist and ophthalmologist involved in evaluating this patient's status both agree that surgery in this case is not advisable.
   a. How will you discuss this with the patient?
   b. During the discussion with the patient, you notice that the patient is becoming very upset, and she looks like she is going to start to cry. How do you handle this?

9. When you are informing a patient of bad news, what cues can you look for to help you determine when the patient is ready to hear further

information? How do you know if a patient is experiencing "information overload"? What signs do you look for in monitoring a patient's response?

REFERENCES

Alpert JS, Wittenberg SM. A Clinician's Companion: A Study Guide for Effective and Humane Patient Care. Boston: Little, Brown, 1986.

Anderson CA. Patient Teaching and Communicating in an Information Age. Albany, NY: Delmar Publishers, 1990.

Blum RH. The Management of the Doctor–Patient Relationship. New York: McGraw-Hill, 1960.

Cohen-Cole SA. The Medical Interview: The Three-Function Approach. St. Louis: Mosby Year Book, 1991.

Herrin S. This patient is going blind: How do you break the news? Review of Optometry 120:47–36, 1983.

Klein SD, Klein RE. Delivering bad news; the most challenging task in patient education. Journal of the American Optometric Association 58:660–663, 1987.

Kübler-Ross E. On Death and Dying. New York: Macmillan, 1969.

Slamovits TL, Macklin R, Beck RW et al. What to tell the patient with optic neuritis about multiple sclerosis. Survey of Ophthalmology 36:47–50, 1991.

ADDITIONAL READINGS

Buckman R. How to Break Bad News—A Guide for Health Care Professionals. Baltimore: The Johns Hopkins University Press, 1992.

Buckman R. Breaking bad news—Why is it still so difficult? British Medical Journal 228:1597–1599, 1984.

Fischer BA. Fine-tuning the message. Optometric Economics 2:13–21, 1992.

Handler G. Remember the person behind the eyes. Optometric Management 24:88–92, 1989.

Litwin MS. Ode to joy. Annals of Internal Medicine 117:337, 1992.

Lowe J, Drasdo N. Patients' responses to retinitis pigmentosa. Optometry & Vision Science 69:182–185, 1991.

Quill TE, Townsend PT. Bad news: Delivery, dialogue, and dilemmas. Archives of Internal Medicine 151:463–468, 1991.

Rodgin SG. Ocular and systemic myasthenia gravis. Journal of the American Optometric Association 61:384–389, 1990.

Shindell S. Psychological sequelae to diabetic retinopathy. Journal of the American Optometric Association 59:870–874, 1988.

6

Building Doctor–Patient Rapport

Doctor–patient rapport refers to the relationship that exists between the doctor and the patient. Ideally, the ultimate relationship is characterized as warm, therapeutic, and conducive to good care. In contrast, clinical encounters sometimes result in anxiety and antagonism. Patients change doctors most frequently because of a doctor's attitudes and lack of good communications (Bennett 1980; Gerber 1989). It is less common for a patient to leave a doctor based on a belief that the doctor is not proficient or competent (Friedman and DiMatteo 1990). Unless a very obvious error is made, patients may have very little basis for judging a doctor's competence; however, they *do* have a basis for judging the quality of the doctor–patient interaction and for evaluating their feelings about the doctor. These latter characteristics are often used by patients as a gauge of the quality of care that they receive. When the doctor–patient interaction is ineffective or negative, it creates an obstacle to the effective delivery of clinical services.

Recommendations for improving doctor–patient rapport will be discussed in this chapter. Use of qualities such as respect, concern, understanding, empathy, and sensitivity are valuable in fostering effective doctor–patient interactions. Transference and countertransference can negatively affect the relationship and recommendations will be explored to deal with these issues. Models of different types of doctor–patient relationships and their advantages and disadvantages will be presented in this chapter (Stewart and Roter 1989; Szasz and Hollander 1956).

TYPES OF DOCTOR–PATIENT RELATIONSHIPS

A common system for analyzing the doctor–patient relationship looks at the spectrum of high and low control, as maintained by the doctor and patient in the relationship (Stewart and Roter 1989). High control is representative of active participation, while low control is characterized by passive involvement or indifference. The four possible relationships (paternalism, default, consumerism, and mutuality) are described in Table 6.1.

Paternalistic Relationship

The paternalistic relationship, in which the doctor holds high control and the patient low control, is the "typical" form of the doctor–patient relationship. In this relationship the doctor "knows all" and the patient comes to the doctor for "divine," magical powers of expertise. Some patients find this type of relationship appealing because it puts the burden of the patient's health on the doctor. For patients with life-threatening and incurable conditions, sharing the burden can be helpful (Stewart and Roter 1989). Characteristically, the patient in this relationship yields to the doctor, and will theoretically follow whatever the doctor says.

Once the patient leaves the doctor's office, however, there is little control of the execution of the doctor's recommendations. If questions or problems arise, patients usually will not call or return to the doctor before they are instructed to do so. They are usually uncomfortable with asking

Table 6.1 Types of doctor–patient relationships

Category Type	Doctor/Patient Control	Description
Paternalistic	Doctor—high control Patient—low control	Doctor characterized as divine, magical "know-it-all"; patient yields to doctor's decisions
Default	Doctor—low control Patient—low control	Lack of continuity of care and absence of active participation by both the doctor and patient
Consumerist	Doctor—low control Patient—high control	Patient views the doctor–patient relationship as a business interaction; relationship often based on distrust and suspicion
Mutuality	Doctor—high control Patient—high control	Active participation and cooperation by doctor and patient; doctor provides education to help patient take increased responsibility for health status

the "omnipotent" doctor questions; there is a minimum of patient feedback. These patients typically take little responsibility for their health care, so they may forget or fail to go for recommended referrals, tests, or consultations.

Many doctors have found this form of interaction to be personally satisfying and gratifying. However, in recent years, this form has been held in disfavor within the health care community because it prevents patients from taking an active role in their health status.

Default Relationship

The interaction in which both the doctor and the patient exhibit low control is the "default" relationship. Both the doctor and the patient are passive with respect to the patient's health and clinical status in this type of interaction. A characteristic example is the patient who rarely visits the doctor and does not follow recommendations. The doctor loses track of the patient when the patient does not return for follow-up care. The theme in this health care relationship is "whatever happens, happens." The lack of continuity of care and the absence of active participation by both the patient and doctor result in less than optimal clinical outcomes.

Consumerist Relationship

The opposite of the paternalistic relationship, the consumerist relationship is characterized by the low control of the doctor and high control of the patient. Although research has indicated that older, less educated patients who are more accepting of authority are more prone to seeking a "paternalistic" doctor–patient interaction, it is believed that younger, better educated, more skeptical patients are more likely to seek a "consumeristic" relationship (Stewart and Roter 1989). This type of patient is often demanding of information and services. The patient in this interaction sees the relationship as a business transaction, and may "shop around" until he or she decides whether to buy. This type of relationship has been criticized because the doctor–patient relationship is based on distrust, suspicion, and skepticism. The limitations within this interaction prevent the doctor from forming what would be a truly therapeutic and helping relationship.

Mutuality Relationship

The mutuality relationship describes an interaction in which the responsibility for the patient's health is a joint venture that is shared by both the doctor and the patient. Both individuals participate actively in this form of interaction, with a relatively even balance of control. The mutuality relationship is currently considered the optimal form of interaction between the doctor and patient because it involves a cooperative collaboration between the two individuals. The doctor has the opportunity to assess the patient's health optimally and to consider appropriate alternatives. Patients take appropriate responsibility in understanding their health status so they can appropriately execute the indicated recommendations. The doctor in this relationship is actively involved in patient education and in negotiating with the patient to develop realistic and therapeutic management plans (see Chapter 7).

SZASZ AND HOLLANDER MODEL

Three similar forms of doctor–patient relationships, associated with characteristic examples of clinical situations, were proposed by Szasz and Hollander (1956). The **activity–passivity model** portrays the doctor as the *provider* of clinical care, and the patient as the *recipient* of clinical care. Like the "paternalistic" model, the doctor is portrayed as the all-powerful figure and the patient as the helpless, inactive recipient of care. For example, patients who are examined under anesthesia or are receiving emergency care for acute trauma may have little power to function actively within the clinical experience.

The **guidance–cooperation model** also emphasizes the dominant, controlling role of the doctor, but gives the patient specific, but limited, responsibilities within clinical care. The doctor guides by providing the directions, and the patient cooperates and complies with the doctor's recommendations.

The **mutual participation model**, most like the mutuality relationship, involves the doctor and patient in a cooperative, collaborative relationship. There is shared responsibility between the doctor and patient and both individuals pursue a common goal of eliminating illness and maintaining health. Management of chronic diseases, such as diabetes, hypertension, and glaucoma, require changes in life styles that can benefit from the mutual participation relationship.

These models can be used to improve the quality of clinical care. Based on the individual's needs, the doctor can determine which model will help build a therapeutic relationship. By listening to patients, understanding their needs and concerns, and identifying the proper level of support needed, the doctor can evaluate how to model and build a relationship that is uniquely suited for each doctor–patient interaction.

Ms. Andrews is a 42-year-old patient with AIDS. She was diagnosed as HIV-positive four years ago, and has had several serious AIDS-related illnesses in the past two years. She comes to the eye doctor complaining of blurred vision. The eye doctor identifies that she has *cytomegalovirus* (CMV) retinitis.

The doctor considers which type of relationship is best with this patient. A mutuality relationship? A paternalistic relationship? One of the other forms? What should the doctor tell this patient about her prognosis?

Discussion:

It is impossible to answer these questions based on the clinical details provided alone. Building an appropriate relationship involves listening to the patient, understanding her needs and concerns, and identifying the proper level of support needed. The patient's needs depend to some extent on her level of acceptance. Is she in denial or shock? Is she angry or depressed? Has she accepted her diagnosis? How is she coping? What is her foundation of support from family and friends?

The emergence of AIDS and HIV disease has resulted in patients who express a much greater interest in participating in clinical decision making. Public education about the therapies and treatments of HIV and AIDS has resulted in more knowledgeable and better educated patients. Consequently, many patients seek a "mutuality" relationship in which the doctor discusses the alternatives, and decisions are made jointly. According to one patient, "If I am going to die, I want to have some control over the rest of my life."

Some patients with serious illnesses view clinical care as more of a "consumerist" affair, searching for a doctor who will do what they desire. These patients can be helped by building a sense of trust, providing education to answer their questions, and giving them adequate opportunities for participation in decision making. When discussing prognosis, the doctor should monitor a patient's response to initial information provided. What follow-up questions does the patient ask? Does the patient appear to desire additional details? What does the patient's nonverbal behavior indicate about the patient's level of understanding, acceptance, and interest? Doctors can be most effective in forming a helping relationship by having the insight to share appropriate information with the patient at the right time, and the flexibility to be responsive to the individual patient's needs at all times. The best recommendations are to listen to a patient's questions, provide adequate patient education, encourage the patient to share concerns openly, and reassure the patient of your continuing support.

TRANSFERENCE AND COUNTERTRANSFERENCE

In addition to applying the models of relationships to each doctor–patient interaction, understanding difficult situations like transference and countertransference can help the doctor improve clinical care.

Transference and countertransference can have significant effects on the doctor–patient relationship. It is not uncommon for doctors and patients to unconsciously "transfer" attitudes and feelings from other relationships onto each other. A doctor who reminds a patient of another person (e.g., a parent or other "authority" figure with similar looks, personality, or social stature) may evoke the same feelings within that patient as the other person. Attitudes that are displaced in this manner can be positive or negative and may not be appropriate for the specific doctor–patient encounter: a patient may be unusually friendly or highly antagonistic toward a doctor. These situations are often difficult for doctors, who cannot understand the basis for a patient's reactions. It is a principle of ethics that doctors and clinical students should not take advantage of patients' feelings of transference. Learning to recognize and handle transference and countertransference can help the doctor manage these situations.

The disparity of power within the doctor–patient relationship may also result in patients who exhibit sexually seductive behaviors. They may see the doctor as an important, powerful, distinguished individual, and they may become attracted to this image. According to Cohen-Cole (1991), sexually seductive behaviors by patients stem from "the grossly unequal power in the doctor–patient relationship and the psychological dependency" that patients have on their health care professionals. He cautions clinical students and doctors "to remember . . . [that] a sexual relationship between a doctor and his or her patient is always an abuse of power in the doctor–patient relationship. This is unethical . . . and exploitative." Managing patients who display seductive behaviors is discussed further in Chapter 14.

Recommendations for Managing Transference

1. When patients respond to clinical situations in an unexplained manner, consider the possibility of transference.
2. To better understand patients' underlying concerns, allow patients the opportunity to express their feelings, and respond supportively. If patients express resistance or antagonism, avoid the temptation of responding in a defensive manner. Defensive reactions often make patients more argumentative and intensify the difficulty between the doctor and patient. Instead, acknowledge the patient's emotional and affective level, address the patient's concerns, and express your interest in providing a safe and supportive environment for the patient.
3. Remember that patients who exhibit sexually seductive behaviors are responding to the disparity of power inherent in the doctor–patient relationship. Recommendations on handling clinical situations in which patients display seductive behaviors are presented in Chapter 14.

Handling Countertransference

Countertransference refers to feelings and emotions that health professionals "transfer" toward their patients. Like transference, countertransference can evoke positive or negative emotions. An impatient elderly patient may remind the doctor of an ailing parent or grandparent, and feelings associated with this family member may be generated toward the patient. Patients who are unkempt or who fall within certain socioeconomic categories may evoke feelings that the doctor has had toward others within these categories. Physically attractive patients may evoke feelings of attraction within the doctor. The ability to recognize countertransference and to return the relationship to an objective professional level can improve clinical care.

Recommendations for Managing Countertransference

1. Doctors must realize that feelings for other individuals are natural, and they should not feel guilty or embarrassed about them; however, they must not act on feelings that are inappropriate, and they must use good judgment in handling these feelings.
2. When they recognize these feelings, the doctor should make sure to maintain an objective, professional relationship.
3. It is especially important to remember the disparity of power inherent in the doctor–patient relationship, and the ethical principle of never taking advantage of that role.

   Ms. Ross is a 79-year-old female who presents to the doctor. She has cataracts and macular degeneration. She reminds the doctor of an elderly grandmother who became very argumentative and dependent on relatives in her later years. Although Ms. Ross is very sweet and undemanding, the doctor responds to her on occasion in a defensive manner. When analyzing this response, the doctor recognizes the existence of countertransference. This enables the doctor to control negative reactions better, and to treat the patient objectively.

BUILDING GOOD DOCTOR–PATIENT RAPPORT

Understanding the different types of doctor–patient relationships and difficult situations like transference and countertransference can help the doctor improve clinical interactions. Understanding the characteristics of successful rapport can also be helpful. These qualities operate actively between doctors and patients throughout the clinical examination.

Doctor–patient rapport begins to develop at the onset of the clinical encounter. A patient's first impression of a doctor can have a significant effect. The value of a smile and a warm handshake when the doctor greets a patient should not be underestimated. The doctor should also be sensitive in using the patient's name when greeting the patient, and frequently thereafter to develop a connection with the patient.

The following qualities are basic to the foundation of good doctor–patient relationships. By being aware of these characteristics, and demonstrating them during clinical encounters, doctors and clinical students can learn to put their patients at ease and develop more effective relationships.

Respect

Treating patients respectfully means accepting them for who they are, and not judging them. Doctors may not agree totally with their patients' beliefs and values, and they may not share their styles of dress, but they can be fully accepting of the patient's identity and priorities.

Concern

Showing concern for a patient involves demonstrating a caring attitude and an interest in the patient's problems and needs. Providing the patient with the doctor's undivided attention during the examination and giving patients adequate time to discuss their questions and concerns are helpful in demonstrating that a doctor is a caring, concerned clinician.

Some doctors have the ability to make each patient feel that he or she is the most important person sitting in the doctor's office. This is a true demonstration of concern and interest in the patient.

Understanding

Conveying an understanding attitude toward the patient shows that the doctor is interested in the patient's concerns and perspectives. Patient orientation, rather than unmitigated problem or doctor orientation, is the hallmark of an understanding health care professional.

Trust

Patients have to trust their doctors to cooperate and comply optimally. Without a sense of trust, patients are often defensive, apprehensive, or evasive. The doctor can start to establish a sense of trust during the encounter by encouraging patients to express their concerns openly.

To be perceived as trustworthy, the doctor must maintain a reputation characterized by a consistent pattern of honesty. Do not tell a patient that a procedure does not hurt if it does; instead, say "You may feel your eye sting for a few seconds after I put this drop in your eye, but the sensation will quickly disappear." Once a patient has reason to question the truthfulness of a doctor, the doctor's future credibility to the patient may be impaired. Remember that children are especially sensitive to their perceptions of whether a doctor is trustworthy and "safe."

Empathy

Empathy is the ability to *understand* the viewpoint of another individual *and* the ability to *communicate* that understanding to the person. Doctors can convey empathy through both verbal and nonverbal cues, and they can benefit greatly by becoming proficient in the skills of empathic listening and responding (see Chapter 3).

Sensitivity

By being sensitive to the patient's concerns, priorities, and feelings, the doctor can orient communications and care to the needs of the patient.

Sincerity

Sincerity involves a genuine, authentic interest in patients, and in the doctor's ability to help them. Patients can usually tell when doctors are sincere and dedicated to their patients. Sincerity is not a measurable, tangible entity but its value in contributing to caring relationships is monumental.

SUCCESSFUL CLINICAL INTERACTIONS

The information presented in Chapters 1 through 6 forms the groundwork for establishing a doctor–patient rapport. Using the skills learned in the previous chapters, such as good listening, nonverbal communication, and supportive communication, the doctor can foster rapport. Understanding the dynamics and characteristics of doctor–patient interactions discussed in this chapter can further improve the doctor's ability to develop a supportive clinical environment. Patients often come to the clinical setting nervous, apprehensive, and anxious. The doctor who puts the patient at ease, physically and emotionally, has taken a large step in developing a helping relationship.

STRATEGIES FOR BUILDING DOCTOR–PATIENT RAPPORT

Establishing and building doctor–patient rapport are essential aspects of delivering clinical care. A patient's satisfaction with the delivery of clinical care is often associated with the quality of the interaction between the doctor and patient.

1. Never, never tell the patient something that you do not absolutely believe to be the truth. Once a patient has reason to question or doubt what the doctor says, the credibility of that health professional may be irreparably tarnished and impaired.
2. *Listen* to your patients (see Chapter 2). Good listening and responding skills are basic elements in building doctor–patient rapport.
3. Be aware of the first impressions that you make on your patients. The first impression that you make on a patient can have a significant impact on your ability to establish and build doctor–patient rapport.
4. Learn the art of putting the patient at ease.
5. Refer to the patient by name at the onset of the examination, and frequently throughout the examination. Referring to a patient by name is a way of building an interpersonal bond.
6. Respond to patients' emotional cues and communications. By attending to the patient's affective needs, the doctor shows a sensitivity and concern for the patient.
7. Learn to handle experiences of transference and countertransference more effectively.
8. Remember to demonstrate and cultivate the seven characteristics of the caring clinician: respect, concern, understanding, trust, empathy, sensitivity, and sincerity.

QUESTIONS FOR THOUGHT

1. Name and describe the different types of doctor–patient relationships. Which do you feel is the most effective form?
2. A patient presents to your office for care. The patient is very subservient, and treats you as the "omnipotent" doctor. Would you encourage this behavior, or would you try and modify the patient's response to you?
3. A patient expresses a "consumerist" attitude, challenging you on why you are doing all of your tests. ("Doc, why do you have to do all these tests, with all this fancy equipment? Health care is so expensive, and the doctors keep you coming back for more tests.") You find that the patient is a glaucoma suspect, and you want the patient to come back for another intraocular pressure measurement and for visual fields. What do you say to the patient?
4. You examine and fit a new patient with contact lenses. You know that as a contact lens wearer, this patient must maintain adequate lens care, and return for periodic follow-up appointments. How would you go about developing a "mutuality" relationship with this patient?

5. You examined a 49-year-old male patient eight years ago. When he returns to you, he tells you that he has not had an eye examination since he came to you last time. You explained to him then, and reexplain to him at this examination, the importance of routine eye care. He says that he goes to doctors only "when something hurts, or when it is absolutely necessary." He adds, "It takes too much time, and I hate to sit behind those instruments." How do you build doctor–patient rapport with an individual who is very resistant to clinical care?

6. Discuss the seven qualities of effective doctor–patient relationships. How do you demonstrate these characteristics to patients?

7. Define transference and countertransference, and give examples of each. Have you had any experiences with these? Explain and describe any experiences that you have had, and how you handled them.

REFERENCES

Bennett I. The patients who got away. Optometric Management October:21–27, 1980.

Cohen-Cole SA. The Medical Interview: The Three-Function Approach. St. Louis: Mosby Year Book, 1991.

Friedman HS, DiMatteo MR. Patient-physician interactions. In Shumaker SA, Schron EB, Ockene JK, eds., The Handbook of Health Behavior Change. New York: Springer, 1990.

Gerber PC. Contact lenses: Refits revival. Eyecare Business July:57–58, 1989.

Stewart M, Roter D. Communicating with Medical Patients. Newbury Park, CA: Sage Publications, 1989.

Szasz TS, Hollander MH. A contribution to the philosophy of medicine. Archives of Internal Medicine 97:585–592, 1956.

ADDITIONAL READINGS

Bernstein L. Interviewing—A Guide for Health Professionals. Norwalk, CT: Appleton-Century-Crofts, 1985.

Comstock LM, Hooper EM, Goodwin JM, Goodwin JS. Physician behaviors that correlate with patient satisfaction. Journal of Medical Education 57:105–112, 1982.

Delbanco RL. Enriching the doctor–patient relationship by inviting the patient's perspective. Annals of Internal Medicine 116:414–418, 1992.

Gregg JR. How to Communicate in Optometric Practice. Philadelphia: Chilton Book Company, 1969.

Guckian JC. The Clinical Interview and Physical Examination. Philadelphia: J.B. Lippincott, 1987.

Innui TS, Carter WB. Problems and prospects for health services research on provider–patient communication. Medical Care 23:521–538, 1985.

Kaplan SK, Greenfield S, Ware JE. Assessing the effects of physician–patient interactions on the outcomes of chronic disease. Medical Care 27:S110–127, 1989.

Korsch BM, Negrete V. Doctor–patient communication. Scientific American 227:66–74, 1972.

Okun BF. Effective Helping Interviewing and Counseling Techniques. Pacific Grove, CA: Brooks/Cole, 1992.

Veatch RM. The Patient–Physician Relation—The Patient as Partner, Part 2. Bloomington, IN: Indiana University Press, 1991.

7

Building Patient Compliance

Compliance (from the Latin *complere*—to fulfill, accomplish) refers to a patient's behavior in following a doctor's recommendations and directions. Patient compliance (or adherence) is a primary component of effective clinical care. In theory, a clinician can do an extensive set of tests—and each test can be performed and recorded impeccably—but unless the patient can be motivated to follow through on the recommendations made, the effectiveness of the doctor may be severely compromised.

Medical researchers have found ways to predict and improve patient compliance (Sackett et al. 1991). Investigations have demonstrated poor prediction of patient compliance by doctors in a wide range of medical specialty areas (Caron and Roth 1968; Mushlin and Appel 1977; Moulding et al. 1970) and in the optometric environment (Kleinstein and Stone 1978). A model for building patient compliance in the eye care environment is presented in this chapter, and strategies for building patient compliance are discussed.

PROBLEMS WITH COMPLIANCE

Noncompliance occurs when a patient fails to follow a doctor's recommendations appropriately. Investigators have estimated that patients remember approximately 50% to 60% of information that doctors give them soon after receiving the recommendations, and about 45% to 55% several weeks later (Coulehan and Block 1987). Understanding and remembering recommendations are primary requirements for compliance.

Problems with compliance may involve taking incorrect doses (too much, or too little) of medications, not taking them at the appropriate times or for appropriate durations, combining medications with other drugs and over-the-counter combinations, not seeking referrals, and not carrying out health-related activities.

Sackett and Snow (1979) found that compliance of patients on short-term medication regimens was approximately 75% for the first few days, but that fewer than 25% of outpatients completed a full 10-day antibiotic therapy regimen. Studies have demonstrated that noncompliance rates of 20% to 30% have been found for curative treatment regimens (e.g., an antibiotic for a particular infection), and 30% to 40% for preventative regimens (e.g., clinical interventions designed to prohibit the onset of disease).

Compliance with medical therapies can be assessed by patient reports, pill and bottle counts, blood and urine tests, mechanical devices, clinical outcomes, and clinicians' estimates. Objective methods (e.g., blood and urine tests, pill counts) tend to report higher levels of noncompliance than patient reports. Blood and urine tests tend to demonstrate higher levels of noncompliance than pill counts.

Clinicians' estimates of patient compliance are frequently poor, and they are often very disparate when compared to other methods of assessment. Caron and Roth (1968) found that 81% of physicians who estimated patient compliance overestimated compliance rates, with assessments that were no more accurate than chance. Mushlin and Appel (1977) found that physicians' predictions of compliance to a medication regimen were incorrect more than half the time, and their predictions in identifying noncompliant patients were incorrect about 75% of the time. Even doctors with long-term relationships with patients showed poor predictions of patient compliance (Gilbert et al. 1980).

Clinical outcomes have sometimes been used to estimate compliance since it is frequently assumed that patients who are more compliant with intervention will do better with treatment. Since there are variabilities in responses to treatment, and differences in an individual's responsiveness at different periods of time, this assumption is not always true.

Coulehan and Block (1987) pointed out that compliance is very doctor-oriented. Compliance, by definition, refers to a patient's *adherence* to a doctor's recommendations. Placing a high value on compliance suggests that a doctor is correct in giving a recommendation, and that a patient is wrong in straying from the advice. This emphasizes the old stereotype of the "all-knowing" doctor, and the patient who is the "recipient" of care (see Chapter 6).

Recent strategies on adherence recommend increased patient participation in designing appropriate management plans. Most problems have a range of patient management options and alternatives. A patient may benefit from a change in a contact lens wearing schedule, contact lens materials, or solution and care regimens. The doctor should consider the possible options for a patient, discuss them with the patient, and consider the advantages and disadvantages of the options for that patient. Anticipating problems in advance, and addressing possible barriers to compliance, can make the clinician more effective in building compliance. Establishing a mutuality relationship by working with the patient to design a reasonable management plan can be most effective (see Chapter 6).

THE HEALTH BELIEF MODEL

The Health Belief Model was designed to help explain under which conditions an individual will carry out health-related behaviors. According to the model, people's behaviors are affected by

1. their perceptions of their susceptibility to a disease,
2. their perceptions of the severity of the disease,
3. the perceived benefits and efficacy of the behavior, and
4. the perceived costs and disadvantages (time, money, convenience, discomfort) of the behavior.

In addition to the factors identified within the Health Belief Model, it is also essential to consider the factors that affect a patient's beliefs on health and illness, and their level of compliance with clinical recommendations (see Chapter 12). Cultural beliefs and "folk healing" practices also affect whether patients will present to doctors with clinical problems, and whether they will comply with clinical recommendations (see Chapter 12). Health care providers should be aware of factors that affect a patient's beliefs and attitudes about clinical treatment (Figure 7.1).

MODEL FOR BUILDING COMPLIANCE

A five-part model for building patient compliance is provided (Table 7.1). In this model, factors that contribute to a patient's behavior in following recommendations are examined.

By considering information about the patient in the first three steps, the doctor can be better prepared to deliver the message in a way that is meaningful to the patient so that it reaches and motivates the patient to follow up. The last part of the model provides strategies that the doctor can use to increase the likelihood of patients' compliance with the doctor's recommendations.

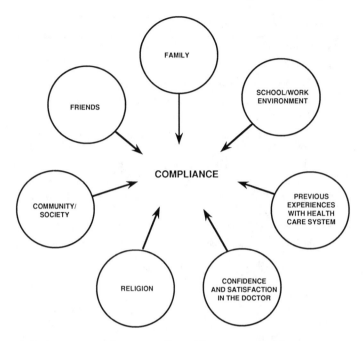

Figure 7.1 Patient compliance is affected by a variety of factors.

Patient Motivation

For each patient, consider what motivates the patient to attend to health care needs. Many patients go to the eye doctor's office because they have signs and symptoms; some understand the importance of routine, periodic eye care, and keep appointments regularly to make sure that their health status is maintained appropriately, even in the absence of symptoms. In each of these cases, the patients have a motivating factor: a *perceived need* for eye care.

Psychologist Abraham Maslow proposed that motivation can be described as a multileveled pyramid, with our most basic needs at its base, and our most sophisticated needs at its apex. In his "hierarchy of needs," Maslow (1954) proposed that a person is not very responsive to higher-level motives (e.g., esteem and self-actualization) until the lower-level motives (e.g., survival and security needs) are met (Figure 7.2). One might expect that health care needs, a low-level motive, would be attended to as a priority by most individuals. Why, then, do many people ignore health concerns and fail to follow through on health care recommendations?

Table 7.1 Building patient compliance

---

1. Patient Motivation

    Consider the following:

    What motivates *this* patient to attend to health care needs?

    Does the patient have a *perceived need* for the recommendations made?

2. Emotional Responses to Health Problems

    Have a sense of the patient's emotional response to being told about a health problem or concern.

3. "Role Modeling" a Patient's Perspectives

    "Role model" the patient—have an understanding of the patient's "personal model of the world" and the perspectives used by this patient in making health care decisions.

4. Delivery of the Recommendation

    The first three steps give the doctor a sense of *how* to deliver the recommendation (e.g., what words to use, emphasis and intonation). The recommendation must be presented in a way that is *meaningful* to the patient. Delivery is a dynamic process, and the clinician who continues to observe the patient, and how he or she responds to the recommendation, can be most effective in reaching the patient—and achieving patient compliance.

5. Strategies of Compliance

    Utilize specific strategies to improve compliance.

The determining factor is often whether a patient has a *perceived need* for health care. If patients perceive that all their health care needs are met, then they will move up to address higher-level goals. If the patient is not aware of an existing health problem, then other needs will probably receive attention. In the absence of signs or symptoms, patients may not realize, acknowledge, or believe that a health problem is present.

If a doctor finds a problem of which the patient was not aware or symptomatic, patient compliance may be challenging to achieve. To increase compliance, the doctor can *build* a perceived need in the patient through several methods, the most prominent of which is patient education.

Demonstration is a particularly strong example of patient education. For example, a doctor who performs accommodative facility testing on a child who responds poorly can create a perceived need for optometric intervention (a program of vision therapy) by explaining to the parents the implications of the responses with respect to the child's classroom difficulties.

By staying aware of a patient's *perceived needs*, and illustrating and demonstrating them when necessary, a clinician can help motivate patients to comply with recommendations.

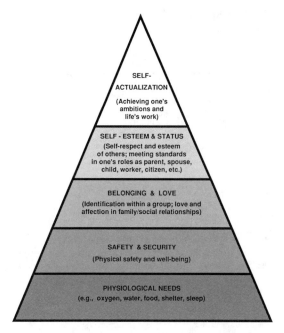

Figure 7.2 Maslow's hierarchy of needs. Individuals are motivated by needs that can be illustrated across a set of levels. A person is not motivated by higher-level needs until the lower ones have been met.

Emotional Responses to Health Problems

A patient's acceptance of a diagnosis can affect whether the recommendations will be followed. Table 5.1 presented a broad range of responses to illness (Kübler-Ross 1969; Blum 1960). These included shock, denial, anger, anxiety, frustration, bargaining, and depression. A spectrum of responses to being told that there is an eye care problem is provided (Figure 7.3). Patients may respond along a continuum, from unresponsiveness to panic, with a wide range of responses in between. The theoretical midpoint, referred to as "responsible attention," would be the response in which a patient responds appropriately and follows a recommendation, with neither excessive concern nor denial.

Some "concern" can actually be a motivating factor for patients to comply and follow up. It is believed that very high levels of anxiety may distract a patient from comprehension, and very low levels may indicate poor levels of patient motivation. Moderate levels of concern appear to be positive factors for patient recall of recommendations.

During the case history and throughout the examination, patients often display their emotional responses to health care concerns. For a patient

Spectrum of responses to being told there is a problem

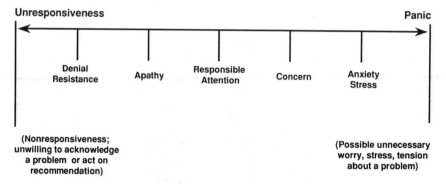

Figure 7.3 Responses to health concerns. Patients respond to news about a health problem with a variety of responses that lie along a continuum ranging from "unresponsiveness" to "panic." The theoretical midpoint, indicated as "responsible attention," is the point at which a patient responds appropriately, with neither excessive concern nor denial.

who is unresponsive and resistant to the presentation of a problem, a stronger case may need to be made to motivate the patient to comply.

Role Modeling the Patient

The art of role modeling the patient, explained in the nursing literature, is described as the process in which the health professional "develops an image and understanding of the client's world—an image and understanding developed within the client's framework and from the client's world" (Erickson et al. 1983).

Each patient's individual perception of the world has a great impact on how a person functions, and on what he or she chooses to do in the world. This perspective, or "frame of reference," is based on a number of factors including current and previous health status, lifetime experiences, background, knowledge, economic status, life style, psychological state, environmental conditions, goals, values, and attitudes.

A doctor who wants to motivate a patient should consider *from the patient's perspective* whether a motivating factor is present. The recommendation can then be presented in a way that is consistent with the patient's needs, desires, and priorities. For example, busy executives may be more willing to invest the time in a badly needed vision therapy program if they realize that an improved visual status will make them more efficient in the many activities at work that involve vision.

Delivering the Recommendation

The first three steps prepare the doctor to deliver the recommendation and give the doctor a sense of *how* to convey the message effectively to a given individual. A most important aspect is that the recommendation be delivered in a way that is *meaningful* to the patient.

As in building patient motivation, to build compliance, the doctor should frame the delivery to the needs of each individual patient. The same recommendation may need to be presented differently to different patients to ensure that each patient will follow up. The strength with which the doctor delivers the recommendation will depend on a number of factors, including the urgency of the action recommended, the patient's motivation, the patient's emotional response characteristics, and the patient's perspective.

To optimize the delivery of the recommendation, the doctor should

- be *clear* about what is recommended;
- be *specific* about what the recommendation entails; avoid vagueness. Say "Rub the contact lens gently with cleaner for about 20 seconds," rather than "rub the contact lens with cleaner." The addition of "20 seconds" and "gently" provides additional information about how the activity is to be done;
- be *conscious* that nonverbal cues (e.g., facial expression, posture, gestures) reinforce the delivery of the recommendation; nonverbal cues that are consistent with the verbal presentation strengthen the delivery of the recommendation;
- present information in "digestible" quantities; avoid "overloading" patients with more information than they can handle at one time;
- utilize repetition to promote understanding and retention of information; repeat important follow-up plans several times or in several different ways;
- give the patient an opportunity to ask questions, *and* use the patient's questions as useful feedback in determining whether the patient has any misconceptions, objections, or resistance to the recommendation. Respond to patient feedback by clarifying the recommendation, correcting any misunderstanding, and calming fears;
- invite the patient to contact you if any additional questions come up.

Some clinicians like to end the delivery of the recommendation by asking for a commitment ("closure") from the patient (e.g., "Can I count on you to make this follow-up appointment?" or "Do you agree that a program of vision therapy can make you more comfortable and efficient at work?").

Appropriate patient education is an important building block toward fostering compliance. For patients to comply, they must understand what is recommended. For specific strategies on patient education, see Chapter 8.

Selecting Compliance Strategies

Many of the strategies for compliance (Table 7.2) involve building a motivating factor within the patient to encourage compliance. Doctors may also
consider combining multiple compliance strategies. For example, a doctor
may provide patient education to explain the importance of a return visit *and*
have the office staff call the patient in advance, to remind the patient of the
appointment. When multiple recommendations are given, it can be very
helpful to provide the patient with a written list of the recommendations so
the patient will remember all of them.

Selecting appropriate compliance strategies is often a question of
"knowing the audience," as discussed in Chapter 1. Knowing the patient can
give the doctor insights into what motivates the patient and what approaches are optimal.

Table 7.2 Compliance strategies

For use in the office
Patient education
Demonstrations to enhance understanding (anatomical models, figures, and diagrams)
Give information in "digestible" quantities
Logic—explain benefits of recommendation to patient
Explain positive outcomes if recommendations are followed
Explain risks of *not* following recommendations
Invite the patient to ask questions
Involve the patient in the determination of management plans
Create a concern or "scare" within the patient
Simplify drug regimens and therapies to make it easier for compliance
Use repetition to enhance memory of recommendations
Ask the patient for a commitment
Enlist the help of accompanying relatives and caretakers (with the patient's permission) in enhancing adherence
Use multiple compliance strategies
For the patient to use at home
Patient literature (printed handouts and diagrams)
Written lists of multiple recommendations to enhance memory
Compliance aids (pill organizers, bottle buzzers)
Staying in contact with the patient
Telephone appointment and compliance reminders
Postcard reminders
Follow-up visits to monitor compliance

A 29-year-old male presents to the eye doctor to be fit for contact lenses. As part of the training in handling and using contact lenses, the doctor teaches him about insertion and removal. He is also taught about cleaning and disinfection. Strategies for working to build compliance with this patient include the following.

1. Explain the components of contact lens care in clear, understandable terms that are easy to comprehend.
2. Explain some of the dangers of *not* adhering to these recommendations, such as corneal abrasions and ulcers, as well as the possible occurrence of epithelial staining, neovascularization, dryness, and ocular irritation. This strategy involves using fear to promote compliance.
3. Use logic to build compliance: Since lenses sit on the eye, it is important to keep them clean and clear to facilitate optimal wearing results.
4. Provide *written* instructions to remind the patient how to carry out the designated recommendations at home.
5. Invite the patient to call the office if any questions come up about the proper use and care of the contact lenses.
6. At each follow-up visit, ask the patient to recall the wearing schedule and cleaning/disinfection routine.

A 47-year-old female is diagnosed with chronic open-angle glaucoma, and is instructed to take glaucoma medications. How can the doctor facilitate optimal compliance with this patient?

1. Use logic to explain the cause of glaucoma and the need to control intraocular pressures.
2. Educate the patient extensively on the method and regimen of instilling glaucoma medications (see Chapter 8). Studies have demonstrated the importance of properly instructing patients on the proper method to apply eyedrops. Even patients who have been using eyedrops as part of glaucoma therapy for awhile have demonstrated difficulty in instilling eyedrops, when tested (Brown et al. 1984).
3. Build the drug therapy regimen into the patient's life style. To help the patient remember to instill eyedrops, associate the treatment with meals or time of day. Instruct the patient to take the medications four times a day, after breakfast, lunch, dinner, and at bedtime.
4. Provide the patient with *written* instructions on drug schedules and follow-up appointments to reinforce directions given in the office.
5. Use fear to reinforce the need to comply by discussing the visual consequences of not adhering.
6. Maintain careful records of directions given to patients with the use of drug charts and control sheets (Fingeret and Schuettenberg 1991; Kowal and Fingeret 1987).

7. Monitor compliance over time by asking the patient at *each* follow-up visit to describe the regimen of drug use and method of instillation of drops.

A 54-year-old female presents to the eye doctor for a routine eye examination. She is totally asymptomatic. The doctor finds that her eyes are healthy, with no binocular problems, no oculomotor problems, and no significant change in her prescription. How can the doctor encourage compliance for follow-up visits in this totally asymptomatic patient?

1. Reinforce the need for continued follow-up care and reassure patients that demonstrating good health-related behaviors is necessary or appropriate, despite the lack of symptoms. Use logic to explain to this patient that many ocular problems occur without symptoms, and that routine care is important to identify these problems.
2. Discuss the recommended date for the next appointment. The patient can be preappointed for the following year, and a written reminder provided for the patient. A postcard or phone call can be used to remind the patient of that examination.
3. Develop a good rapport with the patient to facilitate patient confidence, which in turn will facilitate clinical compliance.
4. Provide the patient with patient literature on the importance of routine eye care.

A 46-year-old male with a history of background diabetic retinopathy presents to the eye doctor. How can the doctor facilitate compliance for routine follow-up care in this patient?

1. Use logic to explain to this patient the importance of routine follow-up care, and the need to identify significant changes at an early stage.
2. Discuss the recommended date for the next appointment. The patient can be preappointed for an appointment in six months, and a written reminder can be given to the patient. A postcard or phone call can be used to remind the patient of that examination. Tell the patient very clearly that if any changes in vision are noticed before that visit, to return right away.
3. Remind the patient to continue to present for routine follow-up care to his internist or diabetologist. Logic and fear can help build compliance for routine eye care and medical care.
4. Earn the trust and confidence of the patient so the patient will be motivated to return for your care as you have directed.
5. Enlist the help of relatives (with the patient's permission) to help the patient remember to return for follow-up care.

A 69-year-old male comes to the eye doctor with a complaint of gradually blurred vision. The doctor identifies that the patient has age-related macular degeneration. The doctor wants to motivate the patient to comply with performing Amsler grid examinations at home on a regular basis, and to return on a regular basis for follow-up care. Strategies for working with this patient include the following:

1. Use logic to explain the diagnosis of age-related macular degeneration, the need for follow-up care, and the importance of daily Amsler grid evaluations.
2. Explain the Amsler grid procedure very carefully so the patient will feel confident in performing it, and will understand the importance of the procedure in monitoring his or her continuing status. (See Chapter 8 for educational objectives for teaching patients about using Amsler grids.)
3. Provide the patient with *written* instruction on performing the Amsler grid procedure, in case questions come up at home.
4. Invite the patient to call the office if any questions occur.
5. Use fear to describe the consequences if the patient does not use an Amsler grid and does not return to the doctor in a timely manner.
6. Send the patient postcards, or make telephone calls, to remind the patient of follow-up appointments.
7. At follow-up visits, ask the patient to describe the Amsler grid procedure, to make sure that it is being performed correctly. Provide corrective comments and feedback, when indicated.

STRATEGIES FOR BUILDING COMPLIANCE

1. Know the factors that influence compliance. Consider the patient's health beliefs, previous experiences with the health care delivery system, and prior compliance record. Also take into account the influence of family, friends, community, religion, and work/school environment.
2. Remember that a patient's satisfaction with a doctor affects compliance. Earn the patient's trust and confidence.
3. Consider a patient's perceived needs and emotional response to a clinical intervention. View the patient's perspective by "role modeling" the patient's response to illness and intervention.
4. Deliver the recommendation in clear terms, avoiding jargon and technical language. Be specific and concise. Present information in "digestible" quantities.
5. In the office, use patient literature and anatomical models to enhance explanations. To encourage compliance, provide literature (handouts and diagrams) for the patient to take home.

6. Give the patient an opportunity to ask questions. A fundamental concept in compliance is if patients do not understand a recommendation, it will be difficult for them to comply.
7. Use logic to explain the importance of a recommendation. Educate the patient about the problem, and the need for action.
8. Use repetition to enhance the patient's memory of information (see Chapter 8, pp. 108–109).
9. Involve the patient in the identification of appropriate management plans. Explain alternatives and allow the patient to participate in the discussion of plans.
10. Decrease patient anxiety by telling the patient what to expect in a supportive manner. Describe positive outcomes resulting from good compliance and explain risks of noncompliance.
11. Obtain closure from the patient by asking for a commitment to follow the doctor's recommendations.
12. Work to establish a perceived need for intervention. If this is ineffective, create a concern within or "scare" the patient to build compliance.
13. Simplify drug regimens and therapies when possible to facilitate compliance.
14. Offer life style applications and help fit recommendations (e.g., glaucoma therapy) into the patient's life style and daily activities to promote a patient's memory of health-related behaviors.
15. With the patient's permission, enlist the help of accompanying caretakers and parents in adherence to recommendations.
16. Use positive reinforcement: acknowledge good compliance habits when they are observed at follow-up visits. To maintain compliance over time, adherence to recommendations should be reinforced.
17. Multiple compliance strategies can be even more effective than a single method. Utilize compliance strategies, patient literature, and compliance aids to assist in building compliance (see Table 7.2).
18. If multiple recommendations are made, provide a written list for the patient for use at home.

QUESTIONS FOR THOUGHT

1. You are caring for a patient who has just been diagnosed with glaucoma. The patient has been instructed to use drops daily to reduce the intraocular pressures.
   a. What strategies can you use to try to build compliance for glaucoma therapy with this patient?
   b. When the patient returns for follow-up care, what information will be available to help you assess the patient's level of compliance?
2. What factors affect a patient's health beliefs?

3. According to the Health Belief Model, what four criteria do patients use in determining whether to carry out health-related behaviors? When all four criteria are not met, what steps can you take to try to improve compliance?
4. When you are determining a management plan for a patient, do you consider the patient's potential compliance? Should a doctor try to consider the patient's potential compliance when choosing a management plan? If you were deciding between two plans, and you felt that one would be slightly better for the patient, but that the patient would be more likely to adhere to the second, which would you choose?
5. Some health care professionals like to use fear as a method of building patient compliance, and some feel that fear is not an appropriate tactic. How do you feel about this, and what are the arguments for both sides?
6. You have examined a 32-year-old female who has an accommodative infacility and a convergence insufficiency. You determine that vision therapy is the optimal strategy to address this patient's symptoms. She is an administrative assistant, and mentions that she does not have a lot of time available to devote to this problem. You want to consider factors that may motivate this patient to comply with your recommendation. How can you "role model" this patient to understand her "model of the world?" How can understanding a patient's perspective in this type of case help you build compliance?
7. You want to initiate a project in your clinical environment to encourage compliance with recommendations for routine eye care. In many cases, patients do not return until they are having a problem. You want to foster compliance in your patient population even in the absence of symptoms. What compliance strategies can you use in your clinical setting to accomplish this task?

REFERENCES

Blum RH. The Management of the Doctor–Patient Relationship. New York: McGraw-Hill, 1960.

Brown MM, Brown GC, Spaeth GL. Improper topical self-administration of ocular medication among patients with glaucoma. Canadian Journal of Ophthalmology 19:2–5, 1984.

Caron HS, Roth HP. Patients' cooperation with a medical regimen. Journal of the American Medical Association 203:922–926, 1968.

Coulehan JL, Block MR. The Medical Interview: A Primer for Students of the Art. Philadelphia: F.A. Davis, 1987.

Erickson HC, Tomlin EM, Swain MP. Modeling and Role Modeling: A Theory and Paradigm for Nursing. Englewood Cliffs, NJ: Prentice Hall, 1983.

Fingeret M, Schuettenberg SP. Patient drug schedules and compliance. Journal of the American Optometric Association 62:478–480, 1991.

Gilbert JR, Evans CE, Haynes RB, Tugwell P. Predicting compliance with a regimen of digoxin therapy in family practice. Canadian Medical Association Journal 123:119–122, 1980.

Kleinstein RN, Stone GC. Helping patients to follow their treatment plans. Journal of the American Optometric Association 49:1144–1146, 1978.

Kowal DK, Fingeret M. A glaucoma control chart. Journal of the American Optometric Association 58:734–737, 1987.

Kübler-Ross E. On Death and Dying. New York: Macmillan, 1969.

Maslow AH. Motivation and Personality. New York: Harper & Row, 1954.

Moulding T, Onstad GD, Sbarbaro JA. Supervision of outpatient drug therapy with the medication monitor. Annals of Internal Medicine 73:550–564, 1970.

Mushlin AI, Appel FA. Diagnosing potential noncompliance. Archives of Internal Medicine 137:318–321, 1977.

Sackett DL, Haynes RB, Guyatt GH, Tugwell P. Clinical Epidemiology, 2nd ed. Boston: Little, Brown, 1991.

Sackett DL, Snow JC. The Magnitude of Compliance and Noncompliance. In Haynes RB, Taylor DW, Sackett DL, eds., Compliance in Health Care. Baltimore: Johns Hopkins University Press, 1979.

ADDITIONAL READINGS

Ashburn FS, Goldberg I, Kass MA. Compliance with ocular therapy. Survey of Ophthalmology 24:237–248, 1980.

Becker MH. Patient adherence to prescribed therapies. Medical Care 23:539–555, 1985.

Dubow BW. Repetition: Key to fostering contact lens compliance. Optometric Management 23:42–45, 1988.

Dubow BW, Walker JS. The concept of compliance. Contact Lens Spectrum 5:45–47, 1990.

Ghormley NR, Ardisson TJ. AOSept lens care system or Opti-Free system? To what extent does patient preference influence compliance? Contact Lens Spectrum 6:35–37, 1991.

Granstrom P, Norell S. Visual ability and drug regimen: Relation to compliance with glaucoma therapy. Acta Ophthalmolgica 61:206–219, 1983.

Kass MA, Gordon M, Meltzer DW. Can ophthalmologists correctly identify patients defaulting from pilocarpine therapy? American Journal of Ophthalmology 101:524–530, 1986.

Kass MA et al. Compliance with topical pilocarpine treatment. American Journal of Ophthalmology 101:515–523, 1986.

Kass MA et al. Compliance with topical timolol treatment. American Journal of Ophthalmology 103:188–193, 1987.

Ley P. Communicating with Patients: Improving Communication, Satisfaction and Compliance. London: Croom Helm, 1988.

MacKean JM, Elkington AR. Compliance with treatment of patients with chronic open-angle glaucoma. British Journal of Ophthalmology 67:46–49, 1983.

Meichenbaum D, Turk DC. Facilitating Treatment Adherence: A Practitioner's Guidebook. New York: Plenum Press, 1987.

8

Patient Education: The Doctor as Teacher

Educating patients is an important aspect of clinical care. Clinical care does not end at the completion of the clinical examination. Doctors must also be effective in teaching patients about what they have found, and what needs to be done. If patients are fit with contact lenses and forget the cleaning and disinfection instructions by the time they get home, what impact will this have on clinical care? The effectiveness of clinical care relies on good patient education.

Health care professionals can educate patients about a wide array of factors including health, illness, diagnosis, and management. By effectively teaching patients, doctors can increase the chances that their patients will comply with clinical recommendations and carry out essential health-related behaviors.

To facilitate adherence to recommendations, patients must understand the five Ws: what should be done, when it needs to be done, who should do it, where it is to be done, and why it must be done. A gap in the comprehension of any of these components may reduce the likelihood that a patient will follow through with a recommendation, or carry it out properly.

The doctor who is involved in patient teaching activities should be familiar with learning domains (Anderson 1990; Redman 1988; Nurse's Reference Library 1987) and learning styles (Ley 1988; Coulehan and Block 1987). Patient-oriented teaching strategies and goals should be developed to maximize patient learning. If patients are to follow up adequately on management plans, doctors must also serve as effective educators to their patients.

LEARNING DOMAINS

Patient education involves three learning domains: the affective, cognitive, and psychomotor domains (Anderson 1990; Redman 1988; Nurse's Reference Library 1987).

Before patients can acquire knowledge about health-related behaviors, they must be mentally ready to learn. It is through the affective learning domain that the doctor attends to the emotional concerns of the patient, and helps the patient attain an emotional "readiness" for learning. Stress, anxiety, and fear can impede the learning process; motivation can support effective learning and achievement. By attending to the patient's affective domain, the doctor can facilitate a greater receptiveness to learning.

Through the cognitive domain, patients learn about the facts and details (e.g., who, what, when, where, and why) of activities that are recommended. They become familiar with the components and requirements of a task. Instructions for vision therapy techniques, contact lens disinfection, and eyelid scrub procedures are examples.

Working with patients in the psychomotor domain helps them reach a physical level of preparation for an activity. Through guided responses, patients learn how to insert and remove contact lenses correctly. Although they may have some initial difficulty in knowing how to hold a contact lens, how to keep the eyelids open, and how to place a contact lens on the eye, repetition and practice help to reinforce the motor patterns that direct the action (see Case 8.1).

Although teaching in the clinical environment frequently emphasizes factual (cognitive) and physical (psychomotor) learning objectives, it is important to realize that unless the patient has reached an emotional readiness to learn, the acquisition of new skills and behaviors may be limited. If a patient is uncomfortable about instilling drops in the eye as part of glaucoma therapy, physical mastery of the procedure will be hampered (see Case 8.2). If a patient is very apprehensive about touching the eyelids, inserting contact lenses will remain difficult.

Within each domain, a task can be learned and internalized on any of several progressively complex levels. A doctor may explain the same technique to different patients in different ways, depending on their learning needs. Understanding a patient's mastery within each of these domains can help the doctor identify appropriate learning goals and strategies (see Cases 8.1–8.5).

TEACHING STRATEGIES

Active Participation

In teaching patients, active participation by the patient is advisable. It is not enough to tell patients to do something, and expect them to go home and do it appropriately. Explanations and demonstrations are helpful, but nothing can replace active participation. Watching the patient insert and remove the contact lenses can enable the health care professional to provide essential feedback that can affect performance. Having the patient use a low vision aid in the doctor's office is essential in identifying possible obstacles to proper use.

Involving Sensory Input

It has been recommended that teaching activities simultaneously involve as many of the five senses as possible. For example, the use of written materials, illustrations, anatomical models, videotapes, audiotapes, slides, and demonstrations can involve sight, sound, and touch. It is believed that the combination of the senses in the teaching process promotes learning by providing stronger sensory learning experiences.

> A 74-year-old male has just been diagnosed as having cataracts. The doctor provides a verbal description to the patient to help educate him about his diagnosis. A model of the eye is used in this teaching session to reinforce the discussion. The model can be used to provide visual and tactual cues.
>
> DOCTOR: Everyone has a lens in the eye. Sometimes the lens becomes cloudy. When this occurs, it is called a cataract. (The doctor strengthens this explanation using the model of the eye. He points to the lens in the eye, explains how it is removed, and how another lens is implanted to replace the original. The visual demonstration enhances the verbal explanation.)

Patients with Disabilities

To be effective, learning programs for disabled patients should take any sensory impairments into consideration. For example, patients with hearing impairments should receive plenty of written materials to facilitate learning. Visually impaired patients should be given extensive verbal descriptions and explanations, and printed materials should contain large print to promote effective use. For further information on working with patients with visual and hearing deficits, see Chapter 13.

Primacy and Recency Effects

When patients must be instructed about several recommendations, content and order of presentation both have an impact on what is learned and remembered. In psychological studies of learning, perception, and memory, it has been demonstrated that primacy and recency effects occur (DeVito 1988, 1990). If a subject who is given a long list of words to remember tends to remember the earlier ones best, then a primacy effect has occurred because the earlier information has carried greater weight than the latter information. If the subject tends to remember the latest information best— that is, the words at the end of the list—then a recency effect has occurred because the most recently mentioned information holds the most weight. It has been found that the beginning or end of a list can hold a significant impact; the material that occurs in the middle tends to get lost more frequently.

Knowledge of these effects can be helpful in determining how to present a case disposition to a patient. Discussions with patients are particularly complex if there are multiple problems, and if the doctor wants a patient to remember a group of recommendations. Primacy effects have been found to be particularly useful in presenting clinical recommendations (Ley 1988; Coulehan and Block 1987).

The first strategy is for the doctor to identify priorities within the management plan and structure the discussion of recommendations with the patient. Having prioritized the actions required, the doctor can structure the discussion with the patient. To take advantage of the primacy effect, the doctor should present the most important recommendation first. This should be the recommendation that has the greatest requirement for prompt and timely attention by the patient. Additional recommendations can be presented in descending order of importance.

Repetition is also an important patient education strategy. Important recommendations should be repeated to reinforce learning. After all recommendations have been discussed with the patient, it is helpful to review the most important ones. This can help capitalize on any recency effects, and can provide an opportunity for clarification. At this point, the patient has had a few minutes to think about the recommendation. Initial doubts or areas of confusion may become evident at this point. It is better to review and clarify at this point than to allow the patient to leave with remaining questions.

A 77-year-old male patient with a history of age-related macular degeneration is examined by an eye doctor. He complains of blurred vision in his left eye, which he has noticed for the past few days. The doctor asks a number of follow-up questions related to this symptom. In addition, two other issues arise during the case history. The patient mentions that his sunglasses are scratched and that he wants a prescription to replace the lenses. The patient also mentions that he is using artificial tears for a dry eye problem. The artificial tears have worked successfully and eliminated any discomfort.

During the examination, the doctor finds that the patient has an area of distortion slightly superior to fixation on an Amsler grid. On performing ophthalmoscopy, the doctor sees a possible area of macular edema, and determines that a fluorescein angiogram is necessary.

The doctor has several recommendations to discuss with the patient during the case disposition. The doctor organizes the patient management plan. To capitalize on primacy effects, the most important recommendation is discussed first: the fluorescein angiogram. Then the other recommendations are discussed in order of importance. (If there is no priority among some recommendations, then the order for these does not matter.) The doctor's plan and order of presentation for discussing management with the patient follow:

1. Discuss the need for the fluorescein angiogram and stress the importance of this test. Tell the patient why the test must be done and what will occur during the procedure.
2. Give the patient a prescription for new sunglasses and tell the patient to have them made at his convenience.
3. Recommend that the patient continue using artificial tears as needed.
4. Repeat the most important recommendation to capitalize on repetition and any recency effects. "As I've mentioned, Mr. Winsler, it's important that we set up an appointment for the fluorescein angiogram right away." The doctor asks an office staff member to offer to call to arrange the appointment for the patient.

As with all patients, the doctor gives the patient plenty of time to ask questions during the discussion.

Understanding the effects of primacy, recency, and repetition can enable the doctor to facilitate maximum retention of essential recommendations.

Providing Written Recommendations

When multiple recommendations are presented, the doctor may choose to provide the patient with a written list of the recommendations. This can help to enhance retention, accuracy, and long-term adherence to the recommendations. Most clinicians present recommendations verbally, but many rarely or never present them in writing. Providing a written list reinforces what has been said and adds a different sense—vision—to the learning experience. As described earlier, it is believed that involving as many senses in the teaching activity as possible is beneficial. Giving the patient a written list involves another dimension. It provides a permanent list of the doctor's suggestions that is not subject to the same compromise in accuracy that reliance on a patient's memory presents.

Check Understanding and Invite Questions

It is helpful to check a patient's understanding of a recommendation by asking him or her to repeat the directions that will be followed. In addition, it is important to provide the patient with an opportunity to ask any questions, or to clear up any areas that are not fully understood. The following example illustrates this point.

DOCTOR: Do you think that you have a good understanding of how you will clean your contact lenses?

PATIENT: Yes, I think I have it pretty straight.

DOCTOR: Can you repeat to me how you will clean them?

PATIENT: When I remove the lens from my eye, I'll put a drop of daily cleaner on the lens and I'll rub it gently for about (patient hesitates).... How long do I rub the cleaner?

DOCTOR: For about 20 seconds.

PATIENT: Right. Then I'll wash the cleaner off with saline solution, and put it in the case with the soaking solution. How am I doing so far?

DOCTOR: Just fine. Keep going.

PATIENT: I'll enzyme the lenses once a week. I think that's it, isn't it?

DOCTOR: Yes, that was very good. I am also going to give you the written directions to take home with you. If you have any questions, you can look at the written directions. Also, please feel free to call our office.

STYLES OF LEARNING

The doctor who is approaching the teaching task should remember that different patients have different styles of learning. Some learn faster than others, and some require a slower presentation of information. Some have more self-confidence, and others require more support. Use of language must also be tailored to the individual's needs.

Personality is another factor affecting learning in the clinical environment. Patients with different personalities communicate and interact with the doctor and office staff differently. These characteristics have to be considered when planning the teaching task.

Visual, Auditory, and Tactual Learners

Patients respond differently to different types of information. Some individuals learn better from auditory input, some from visual input, and some from tactual input. In many cases, one modality reinforces the other, with one sense having the major influence on learning. When explaining a diagnosis, models of the eye and anatomical pictures can be used to combine auditory and visual modalities. Effective doctors are skillful in recognizing a patient's preferred sensory modality. The best teaching presentation is one that involves a combination of sensory modalities, with emphasis on the patient's preferred one.

In learning about contact lens insertion and removal, some patients may be most responsive to a visual demonstration, some may be most responsive to a verbal description that accompanies the demonstration, and some may be unresponsive until they get to touch the lenses and try it themselves (tactile input). All patients must practice contact lens insertion and removal when they are newly fit, but some require more visual and verbal instruction than others before they understand and master the process.

Global and Linear Learners

Some patients learn techniques by studying each part, step by step, until they learn the entire procedure. This is a linear approach to learning. Others learn better by looking at the overall objective—the endpoint—and then considering the steps in relation to the "finished product." This is a global approach, and is characterized by an individual who learns best by looking at the whole gestalt of an activity.

The patient learning to insert contact lenses may be a linear learner, concentrating on the details of each step, or a global learner, focusing on the final goal of lens insertion.

STRATEGIES FOR PATIENT EDUCATION

Redman (1988) points out that patient education is a process of communication. The following guidelines can be helpful in designing and selecting productive teaching strategies.

1. When approaching a patient education task, evaluate the patient's "readiness" for learning, and styles of learning, using the following categories:
   a. speed of learning,
   b. use of language,
   c. personality styles,
   d. affective, cognitive, and psychomotor learning domains,
   e. preferences for visual, auditory, and tactual input, and
   f. preferences for linear and global information.
2. In planning teaching sessions:
   a. use techniques that reflect a knowledge of the patient's preferences and learning styles, as described above,

b. use teaching techniques that involve as many of the senses as possible (e.g., visual, verbal, and tactile input),

c. use repetition to reinforce learning,

d. provide written instructions that a patient can take home, to reinforce what has been learned in the office,

e. require active participation by the patient. Do not just describe what patients should do. Let them try home vision therapy techniques before you let them leave. Let them do an Amsler grid evaluation in front of you, as they would do it at home, and

f. invite questions and check understanding by asking a patient to repeat the procedure or regimen that will be followed.

3. When recommendations are discussed with a patient, remember to take advantage of primacy effects in patient discussions by stating the most important information first.

4. Repetition should also be utilized in patient education tasks.

5. When providing patient education, avoid condescending statements and attitudes. Never attempt to impress patients with long, complicated words and terms. This would likely result in miscommunication, and it does little in the way of building doctor–patient rapport.

6. Patient education should always involve follow-up questions at subsequent visits to ensure patient recall and accuracy. Do not assume that a patient is cleaning contact lenses appropriately, or instilling eyedrops using the appropriate schedule, unless you ask.

7. Always provide instructions respectfully. Rushing and impatience are deterrents to the educational setting. Remember that the patient may be nervous, worried, and overwhelmed. The caring patient educator is more likely to create a facilitative learning environment.

Case 8.1

Patient: 34-year-old male, new contact lens wearer.

Teaching Objective: Insertion and removal of contact lenses

A doctor dispenses a first pair of contact lenses to a 34-year-old male. In educating him about insertion and removal of the lenses, the doctor monitors his affective, cognitive, and psychomotor domains. At the beginning, he expresses some concern about touching his lids. "I feel really squeamish about this," he tells the doctor. "I don't like touching the area around my eyes." The doctor responds in the affective domain, assuring him that this is normal in the beginning, and that he will probably feel more comfortable as he practices. The doctor discusses the steps of contact lens insertion, describing the components of the activity. This is the cognitive domain. Then the doctor shows him how to hold the lens on his finger, and how to hold his lids open with his other fingers. The doctor provides him with feedback as he practices. This is the psychomotor domain. Learning objectives for this patient are presented below. Monitoring the patient's progress and mastery within each of the domains guides the doctor in how to provide effective feedback to the patient, and how to proceed with the learning task.

Learning Objectives

Affective Learning Domain

1. The patient demonstrates at least a minimally acceptable level of comfort in touching the area around the eyes and eyelids, adequate for learning to insert and remove contact lenses.
2. The patient demonstrates an adequate level of confidence in performing the steps of insertion and removal before he is allowed to take the lenses home.

Cognitive Learning Domain

1. The patient can explain the steps involved in inserting and removing contact lenses.
2. The patient can identify a problem when it occurs (e.g., if the lens is turned inside out, or if the lens feels uncomfortable when it is inserted) and knows what to do.
3. The patient understands that once the contact lens is removed, there are directions for cleaning and disinfection. (A separate set of learning objectives can be designed for contact lens cleaning and disinfection.)

Psychomotor Domain

For insertion:

1. The patient prepares the proper equipment (e.g., contact lens case, solutions) and identifies a work area.
2. The patient is able to place the contact lens on the index finger, and hold the eyelids open in preparation for insertion.
3. The patient knows how to position the lens on the eye.

For removal:

1. The patient prepares the proper equipment (e.g., contact lens case, solutions) and identifies a work area.
2. The patient is able to hold the eyelids open, slide the contact lens off the cornea onto the conjunctiva with the index finger, and grasp the lens between the index finger and thumb for removal.
3. The patient knows to proceed to steps for contact lens cleaning, disinfection, and storage.

Discussion

Patients who are newly fit with contact lenses must learn to insert and remove their lenses. This often takes excessive time and effort, with patients frequently expressing anxiety and frustration. Identifying learning objectives and monitoring the patient's mastery within each of the domains can make this process more effective and efficient for both the doctor and patient.

Case 8.2

Patient: 59-year-old female, recently diagnosed with chronic open-angle glaucoma.

Teaching Objective: Instilling glaucoma medications

A 59-year-old female is diagnosed with chronic open-angle glaucoma in her right eye, and is told to start using drops to reduce the intraocular pressures in that eye. The doctor presents the patient with a prescription. This patient must deal with the emotional pressure of accepting a new disease entity and she must take on the responsibility of putting drops into her eyes.

The patient returns to the doctor in a month. The doctor finds that the intraocular pressure is not reduced. On further questioning, the doctor ascertains that the patient is somewhat uncomfortable in administering the drops, and she is not sure that she is getting them in her eye fully. The doctor realizes that the patient should have been taught to instill the eyedrops in her eye.

Learning Objectives

Affective Learning Domain

1. The patient demonstrates that she is emotionally ready to touch areas around the eyes and eyelids to instill the eyedrops.
2. The patient displays a personal commitment and motivation to adhere to the regimen of instilling drops.

Cognitive Learning Domain

1. The patient understands the nature of glaucoma (increased intraocular pressure in the eye) and the reason she must instill drops in her eyes regularly.
2. The patient can describe the steps involved in instilling drops into the eye.
3. The patient can describe the appropriate protocol, as directed by the doctor (e.g., one drop daily, twice a day, four times a day, etc.).
4. The patient demonstrates an understanding of the importance of returning to the doctor regularly, as directed, to evaluate the effectiveness of therapy.

Psychomotor Learning Domain

1. The patient grasps the bottle of eyedrops in preparation for instillation.
2. The patient demonstrates making a pocket in the lower cul-de-sac by grasping the lower eyelid and pulling it away from the eye.
3. The patient knows where to hold the bottle in relation to the eye.
4. The patient looks upward when the eyedrop is released, and holds the eye open appropriately to facilitate instillation of the drop.
5. The patient avoids touching the tip of the bottle to the eye or eyelid area.
6. The patient holds the eyelid open without blinking immediately after instillation, and then closes the eye for about three minutes. Note: Two more goals can be added to patients' learning objectives, as appropriate.
7. If the patient is told to take more than one drug at a time, she waits at least five minutes before instilling the next drop.
8. The patient demonstrates nasolacrimal occlusion, to reduce systemic absorption.

Discussion

This case demonstrates the need to discuss methods of intervention adequately when they are initiated. The doctor who is caring for this patient should make sure that the patient understands how to carry out the recommended activity. If the doctor just gives her a written prescription, and ignores any discussion on how to instill the drops, the patient may administer them unsuccessfully; if the drop does not get into the eye adequately, it will not attain its optimal effectiveness.

The doctor goes over proper instillation procedures with the patient. At her next visit, the pressures are reduced adequately. This case illustrates that appropriate patient education is essential in obtaining favorable therapeutic results.

Even patients who have been on glaucoma medications for awhile have difficulty instilling drops. A study found that 13% of glaucoma patients already using eyedrops were unable to place drops in their eyes appropriately, and that 80% of them failed to maintain sterility of the bottle during application (Brown et al. 1984). Proper method and understanding of regimen should be checked not only at initiation of therapy, but also at follow-up visits.

Case 8.3

Patient: 19-year-old male, diagnosed with blepharitis.

Teaching Objective: Performing eyelid scrub procedures

A 19-year-old male, complaining of itchy eyes, is diagnosed as having blepharitis. The doctor recommends eyelid scrubs to be performed twice daily, in the morning and evening. As with the patient in Case 8.2, this patient must also become comfortable in approaching and touching the lids.

The doctor instructs the patient on the process of diluting baby shampoo and sweeping gently across the eyelid margins. This is the cognitive content. The doctor gives the patient an instruction sheet to take home with him in case there are any questions.

Learning Objectives

Affective Learning Domain

1. The patient demonstrates that he is emotionally ready to touch areas around the eyes to perform eyelid scrub routine.
2. The patient demonstrates an adequate level of comfort and confidence in carrying out the steps of eyelids scrubs.

Cognitive Learning Domain

1. The patient knows how to dilute baby shampoo with water.
2. The patient can describe how to apply the diluted shampoo along the lid margin with a cotton swab or cloth. (The patient knows to stay at the lid margin, and not to go inside the eye.)
3. The patient knows to return to the doctor if the lids remain irritated, or get worse.

Psychomotor Learning Domain

1. The patient can describe the materials that need to be prepared for eyelid scrubs (baby shampoo, warm water, a cup to make mixture, a cotton swab or a cloth).
2. The patient correctly demonstrates how to administer the baby shampoo along the lid margin: gently moving the cotton swab sideways, not pressing too hard to irritate the lid area.

Discussion

In most cases, doctors leave the psychomotor dimension of eyelid scrubs, in which patients actually practice the procedure, to be handled at home. This can be a disadvantage when patients do not attain a readiness on their own, or when they do not perform the steps of the procedure correctly. When doctors are confident that the psychomotor component of a task can be handled appropriately by the patient at home without extensive training, they are less likely to take extensive time with supervised instruction. When they make this decision, they should always remind the patient to call or return if they have any questions about the procedure.

Case 8.4

Patient: 69-year-old female, with hypertensive retinopathy.

Teaching Objective: Learning to use a low vision aid (hand magnifier)

A 69-year-old female, with long-standing hypertensive retinopathy, has experienced significantly reduced visual acuity. The doctor has discussed the use of the low vision aids with the patient and has determined that a hand magnifier is the best option for this patient.

Learning Objectives

Affective Learning Domain

1. The patient accepts that her vision is reduced as a result of long-standing hypertensive retinopathy, and that this reduction is irreversible.
2. The patient demonstrates an understanding that the low vision aid can help improve her vision, but that it will not restore her vision to the way it was before the impairing condition.
3. The patient can explain that her vision will be different from what she was used to, and that field of view, size of letters, working distance, and lighting requirements are different from previous visual conditions.
4. The patient recognizes that the eye doctor and office staff are available to provide assistance and answer any questions that she may have.

Cognitive Learning Domain

1. The patient demonstrates an understanding of her low vision condition and the need for a low vision device.
2. The patient can describe proper working distance for the hand magnifier.
3. The patient can describe the field of view with the hand magnifier.
4. The patient can describe how to manipulate the hand magnifier and reading material to obtain successive views of printed material.
5. The patient can describe the proper lighting conditions.

Psychomotor Learning Domain

1. The patient demonstrates that she can hold the hand magnifier steady (e.g., without a hand tremor or shake).
2. The patient demonstrates arranging proper lighting.

3. The patient demonstrates holding the reading material and the hand magnifier at the appropriate distances.
4. The patient demonstrates moving the hand magnifier over printed material to obtain successive views.

Discussion

Affective concerns and inadequate psychomotor preparation often present obstacles to a patient's success with low vision aids. Learning objectives that are planned carefully within these domains can improve the adaptation process.

Case 8.5

Patient: 61-year-old male, with age-related macular degeneration.

Teaching Objective: Learning to use an Amsler grid for home monitoring

A 61-year-old male has recently been diagnosed with age-related macular degeneration. The doctor instructs the patient on using an Amsler grid at home.

Learning Objectives

Affective Learning Domain

1. The patient demonstrates an understanding of his retinal problem, and the need to monitor any changes with an Amsler grid.
2. The patient demonstrates a "readiness" to learn to use the Amsler grid.
3. The patient demonstrates a commitment and motivation toward using the Amsler grid at home regularly.
4. The patient displays adequate comfort in handling the Amsler grid and performing the procedure.

Cognitive Learning Domain

1. The patient explains the nature of his visual problem (age-related macular degeneration) and the reason that home monitoring is necessary.
2. The patient describes the proper conditions for performing the Amsler grid evaluation: monocular, wearing the appropriate near correction, proper lighting, holding the grid at 13 inches. The patient also mentions the importance of maintaining fixation on the central dot throughout the test.
3. The patient explains that Amsler grid procedure should be performed daily.

4. The patient describes what to look for routinely on the Amsler grid: all four corners present, any wavy or distorted lines, any boxes missing, any boxes of irregular size.
5. The patient demonstrates an understanding that he knows to call the doctor and seek care immediately if he notices any changes in his Amsler grid observations.

Psychomotor Learning Domain

1. The patient demonstrates that he is able to prepare the appropriate materials for performing the Amsler grid routine: reading glasses, occluder for one eye, the Amsler grid.
2. The patient demonstrates that he holds the Amsler grid at 13 inches, wears his reading glasses, and observes the grid monocularly.
3. The patient switches the occluder over the first eye to test the second eye.

Discussion

Although the Amsler grid is a very important clinical tool, patients often acknowledge limited compliance at follow-up visits. Appropriate preparation and training can enhance performance of this technique.

QUESTIONS FOR THOUGHT

1. Describe the three learning domains involved in patient education. Why is each essential for effective patient learning?
2. For the following patients, how would you design active training programs?
    a. Teaching a patient with low vision to use a hand magnifier.
    b. Teaching a patient to clean and disinfect contact lenses.
    c. Teaching a patient who has just been diagnosed with glaucoma to put drops into the eyes.
3. You are caring for a 79-year-old patient with age-related macular degeneration. You have provided her with an Amsler grid; however, you are not confident that she will remember how to do it, and that she will do it daily. She mentioned several times during your examination that her memory is getting poorer. What steps can you take to ensure that she will use the Amsler grid properly, and that she will remember to do it on a regular basis?
4. Design a training program to teach an adult patient to insert and remove contact lenses. How does your training program address the patient's learning dimensions?

5. One of your patients is a 7-year-old child who is a refractive amblyope. You are going to fit her for a contact lens in the amblyopic eye. The other eye does not require any correction. How would you prepare this child, and her family, to use the contact lens? How would this be different from teaching an adult about contact lens insertion and removal?
6. You have examined a patient and you have to make multiple recommendations. What patient education strategies can you use to enhance the probability that this patient will remember all of them?
7. How can styles of learning and personality types affect a patient's understanding and retention of clinical recommendations?

REFERENCES

Anderson CA. Patient Teaching and Communicating in an Information Age. Albany, NY: Delmar Publishers, 1990.

Brown MM, Brown GC, Spaeth GL. Improper topical self-administration of ocular medication among patients with glaucoma. Canadian Journal of Ophthalmology 19:2–5, 1984.

Coulehan JL, Block MR. The Medical Interview: A Primer for Students of the Art. Philadelphia: F.A. Davis, 1987.

DeVito JA. Human Communication—The Basic Course. New York: Harper & Row, 1988.

DeVito JA. Messages—Building Interpersonal Communication Skills. New York: Harper & Row, 1990.

Ley P. Communicating with Patients: Improving Communication, Satisfaction and Compliance. London: Croom Helm, 1988.

Nurse's Reference Library. Patient Teaching, 1987.

Redman BK. The Process of Patient Education. St. Louis: C.V. Mosby, 1988.

ADDITIONAL READINGS

Bernstein L, Bernstein RS. Interviewing—A Guide for Health Professionals. Norwalk, CT: Appleton-Century-Crofts, 1985.

Gessner BA, Armstrong ML. Patient Teaching. The Nursing Clinics of North America. Philadelphia: W.B. Saunders, 24:583–693, 1989.

Hubler RS. Cataracts: Telling it like it is. Optometric Economics 1(9):24–28, 1991.

Kroeger O, Thuesen JM. Type Talk: The 16 Personality Types That Determine How We Live, Love and Work. New York: Bantam Doubleday Dell, 1988.

Ley P, Spelman MS. Communicating with the Patient. London: Staples Press, 1967.

Lave J, Wenger E. Situated Learning: Legitimate Peripheral Participation. Cambridge: Cambridge University Press, 1991.

Zimmerman TJ, Zalta AH. Facilitating patient compliance in glaucoma therapy. Survey of Ophthalmology 28:252–257, 1983.

Zimmerman TJ, Ziegler LP. Successful topical medication: Methodology as well as diligence. Annals of Ophthalmology 16:109, 1984.

9

Good Recordkeeping

Good recordkeeping is a professional responsibility. It is believed that good records can facilitate effective clinical decision making (Dick and Steen 1991; Weed 1968). Over time, effective records can improve continuity of care. Records that reflect good care can also help to protect doctors in the event of malpractice claims (Classe 1989a,b,c; Classe et al. 1989; Classe and Alexander 1988; Harris and Dister 1987). Clinical care is not limited to performing tests and identifying management plans. All parts of the clinical examination must be adequately documented.

Clinical recordkeeping should include documentation of the case history, clinical findings, patient management plans, and all patient communications. Ultimately, the record should preserve as many of the details and events of the examination as possible. Characteristics of the problem-oriented medical record, suggestions for note-taking during the clinical interview, and benefits to clinical care will be addressed in this chapter.

EFFICIENT RECORDKEEPING

Good recordkeeping is characterized by records that are comprehensive, accurate, well organized, legible, and accessible. Records should consist of a thorough and accurate report of all clinical findings and test results. Doctors should strive to make the record reflect the events of the examination. Ideally, someone reviewing the record should be able to reconstruct the examination as closely as possible.

Records that are well organized can facilitate the clinical thinking process. They can make the process of record review easier for the doctor, office staff, or any possible external sources.

Good records provide both short-term and long-term benefits. Changes in clinical results over time may reflect a variety of clinical problems. Good recordkeeping over time improves continuity of care.

A 59-year-old female presents for a routine eye examination. She has no symptoms. She has no history of ocular disease, although her father has cataracts and glaucoma. Best corrected visual acuities are 20/20 in each eye, at distance and near. Ocular health tests include the following results for the patient's cup-to-disc ratios and tonometry findings:

Direct Ophthalmoscopy:
OD: cup:disc ratio 0.40
OS: cup:disc ratio 0.30

Tonometry (applanation):
OD: 21, 21
OS: 20, 19

In isolation, the above results may appear normal. The doctor looks back at previous records. The patient was in once before, two years ago. The results for similar tests were as follows:

Direct Ophthalmoscopy:
OD: cup:disc ratio 0.25
OS: cup:disc ratio 0.30

Tonometry (applanation):
OD: 21, 20
OS: 19, 20

Although the finding of 0.40 for the cup-to-disc ratio is usually not suspicious, the increase from 0.25 from the previous examination makes the doctor question the events. The patient returns the following morning for a follow-up examination including ophthalmoscopy, tonometry, and baseline visual fields. The cup-to-disc ratios are still 0.40 in the right eye and 0.30 in the left eye.

Tonometry findings at this examination are
OD: 26, 24
OS: 21, 20

The visual field examination reveals no defect in the left eye; however, a small superior-temporal arcuate defect in the right eye, consistent with early glaucomatous changes, is identified. The cup-to-disc ratios of 0.40 and 0.30 alone would probably not have sparked further investigation. An early and timely interpretation of the patient's status is made possible, with the help of previous records.

FILING RECORDS

The filing system that is used to maintain records should also be considered an important component of the recordkeeping process. If a record cannot be found, and if records are frequently misfiled and lost, then the records are not attaining their optimum usefulness. Many clinicians can identify with the experience of stalling a patient in the reception room while the office staff furiously searches for a patient's record. In addition to being complete, well organized, and legible, good records must be accessible to be useful.

PROBLEM ORIENTATION

The Problem-Oriented Medical Record (POMR), developed by Dr. Lawrence Weed (1968, 1969), was designed to improve the process and quality of clinical recordkeeping. This system has also been applied, and used extensively, in optometry (Barresi and Nyman 1978; Sloan 1978; London et al. 1981).

The POMR consists of four parts: the data base, the problem list, the plan, and progress notes. The data base is composed of two parts: the minimum data base and the problem-specific data base. The minimum data base consists of data that are collected on all patients. The problem-specific data base includes clinical findings that address a patient's individual concerns and problems.

Two types of problem lists are used: a working problem list and a master problem list. The working problem list is found at the end of each examination. It consists of a summary of the patient's diagnoses and problems at that examination. The working problem list is usually accompanied by a correspondingly numbered listing of management plans. An advantage of the coordination of the problem and plan lists is that with this system it is less likely that a problem will be forgotten or overlooked when the plans are determined. The master plan is generally found at the *front* of a patient's record. It provides the doctor with an overview of the patient's problems over time. The master plan has been referred to as a "table of contents" of the record (Barresi 1984).

The problem list should reflect the doctor's highest level of understanding. When a diagnosis is known, it is this term that is listed. When the diagnosis is not certain, the problem can be described by the clinical findings or symptoms that are known. Appropriate management plans can then be presented to outline the process for differential diagnosis.

Clinicians should refrain from listing tentative diagnoses in the problem list. Patients tend to get labeled once diagnoses are written on the record, and labels tend to "stick" with patients, even if a tentative diagnosis is ruled out; therefore, it is important to avoid listing tentative diagnoses on the problem list. Possible clinical entities followed by question marks should also be avoided. Problems should be documented at a clinician's highest level of certainty. Tests required to confirm or rule out possible clinical entities can be listed under the management plan, and the doctor's thinking process can be outlined in this section.

Progress notes, composed of four parts, are often referred to by the acronym SOAP (subjective, objective, assessment, plan). Subjective notes are composed of information provided by patients regarding their symptoms, problems, or concerns. Objective notes include the doctor's clinical findings from the examination. The assessment is the doctor's evaluation and determination of the patient's problem or problems. The plan presents the doctor's management strategy and plans for the patient.

The POMR has been criticized at times as time consuming, but the advantages of the system are very easy to understand. The records are well organized, logical, and structured. Continuity of care is enhanced. When used appropriately, the POMR can help contribute to the quality of care provided in the office.

LEGAL ISSUES IN RECORDKEEPING

It has been said that "If it's not written in the record, it wasn't done." In legal cases, the doctor's record is used to establish the set of tests that was done at each visit and the results found. If a test is not recorded, it is assumed that the test was not done. Even if the doctor did a test, and remembers the result, there is no way of proving that it was done unless it is listed on the record.

Malpractice cases invariably involve questions of credibility between the doctor and patient (Scholles 1986). Only by comprehensively documenting the proceedings of the examination can the doctor demonstrate with authority what occurred. Even if the care was appropriate, doctors can be disadvantaged by records that are inadequate and illegible. Documentation of data, changing entries, and recording patient communications are important legal considerations in recordkeeping.

DOCUMENTATION OF CLINICAL DATA

The general rule for recording data is that documentation should be comprehensive, accurate, well organized, and legible. Standard abbreviations within the field can be used, but a doctor's personal abbreviations or shortcuts should be avoided. OD and OS are readily recognized as right and left, respectively; NCT in the space for tonometry is similarly understood as noncontact tonometry. Unrecognized abbreviations or terms can be questioned at a later date, and should not be used.

Results of clinical tests should be recorded using raw data, not just interpretations such as "normal," "negative," or "within normal limits." The recording of WNL (within normal limits) is frequently "translated" humorously as "we never looked." "Within normal limits" is an interpretation of data; the actual numbers found on ophthalmoscopy or tonometry are the findings that should be recorded. The reason for this is that if a question ever arises, "within normal limits" provides no way of telling what the actual data were. A cup-to-disc ratio of 0.40 for an individual is generally considered normal, but if that patient had a cup-to-disc of 0.25 at a previous examination (see page 122), the doctor may not consider that "normal" anymore. Actual findings should be recorded for all clinical tests. Interpretations and management strategies can be found in the problem and plan lists, respectively.

ALTERATION OF RECORDS

Record alterations can be interpreted as deceptive attempts to evade liability; consequently, any changes made to a record must be handled very carefully. When the doctor wants to change an entry in the record, a single line should be used, and the doctor should date and sign (or initial) the change. Rather than obliterating what was written, the single line indicates that the information is unintended, but the original entry is not permanently lost. It is also helpful to list the reason for the change. Figure 9.1 demonstrates examples of acceptable changes.

Always try to record entries properly the first time. Avoid making entries that look like alterations. When changes are necessary, they should be carried out in a timely manner. Once a record is called in question for litigation, the doctor should *never* attempt to modify or add documentation. Regardless of whether the doctor is innocent or guilty, altering the records can severely detract from a doctor's defense.

CONSULTATIONS AND REFERRALS

When patients are referred to other doctors, consultations and referrals should be appropriately documented. The more specific the referral, the better (Classe 1989a). Referring the patient to a doctor by name is better than making a general referral to any practitioner within a specialty area. It is also preferable to call for the appointment from your office, and make the

```
Record # 11245
```

Visual Acuity

Distance: OD ~~20/30~~ 20/25 *eee 9/27/92 Recorded wrong line by mistake, initially.*

OS 20/20

Near: OD 20/20

OS 20/20

```
Record # 11752
```

Tonometry

T(AP)

T_NCT

OD ~~18~~ 16 *eee 9/30/92*

OS ~~16~~ 18 *Reversed results on initial recording.*

Time 10:15 A.M. Drop Fluress

Lid Held? Y (N)

```
Record # 12155
```

Lensometry

OD −5.00 −1.50 x ~~90~~ 180 *eee 10/1/92 Made an error in recording axis.*

OS −7.00 −2.00 x 90

Figure 9.1 Examples of modifications to records. Note that the original entries are crossed out with a single line, leaving the original entry readable. Changes are initialed and dated. A reason for each change is provided.

appointment right away. Then the full entry can be made on the patient's record:

> Referred to Dr. Dayton for Fluorescein Angiography
> Appointment 2/1/94, 10:45 A.M.

If patients reject your attempt to call for an appointment, and prefer to check their schedule and call themselves, this should be documented:

> Referred to Dr. Mattora for Neurology Work-up.
> Patient rejected our offer to call for appointment—wants to check calendar and call on her own.
> Gave Dr. Mattora's name, phone number, and address.

The record should always indicate the reason for the referral and plans for follow-up. To facilitate successful referrals, the patient should be aware of why a referral is necessary (see Chapter 10). If a referral letter is sent to the doctor explaining what services are required, a copy of the letter should be kept and attached to the patient's record. Reports from the consulting doctor should be attached to the record. Phone calls to assess compliance with recommendations for referrals and consultations should also be documented.

PATIENT COMMUNICATIONS

Since it is believed that gaps in doctor–patient communications result in a large proportion of clinical malpractice litigation (Kraushar 1992; Scholles 1986), it behooves the doctor to spend adequate time with the patient providing explanations, and answering questions, and documenting what has been discussed. The doctor–patient interaction is so important that recommendations for improved communication skills for doctors have been referred to as "malpractice prophylaxis" (Cormier et al. 1986).

When patients cancel appointments, or do not show up for a visit, this information should be recorded on a patient's record. Phone calls, letters, or postcards advising the patient to reschedule should also be documented.

It is important to record indications of patient noncompliance. If a patient reports having worn contact lenses longer than the recommended wearing schedule, this should be documented. The patient should be warned of the risks and this should be recorded. Documenting noncompliance can be valuable evidence in the event of litigation.

Patient education should also be recorded. It is particularly important to warn patients of the effects of pharmacological agents used for dilation and cycloplegia, and to record these precautions.

COMMUNICATIONS WITH CONTACT LENS WEARERS

Contact lenses are involved in a large percentage of optometric malpractice cases (Classe 1989a; Classe et al. 1989). This emphasizes the importance of informing patients adequately about appropriate procedures for using contact lenses, and potential risks and complications.

As a result of the voluminous information that must be given to contact lens patients, and the increase in contact lens-related malpractice claims, many practitioners have been using preprinted forms for their contact lens patients. These forms usually include details on fees, refund policies, and required follow-up visits. Obligations of the contact lens wearer, including the need to care for lenses properly and present for regular follow-up care, should be included. All communications concerning contact lens care should be carefully recorded. (Some doctors use a separate form to advise patients about the cleaning and disinfection procedures, and recommended solutions.)

Written forms can also help maintain documentation of informed consent, in which patients are advised of the risks, benefits, and alternatives to contact lens wear, and the probability of success. It is advisable to include a statement that there is no guarantee that the patient will be a successful contact lens wearer (Classe 1989a). There is usually a statement at the end that the patient has read the agreement and understands the contents. The patient is asked to sign and date the form, and a witness is asked to sign. The original is kept in the patient's record, and a copy is provided for the patient.

PROVIDING INFORMATION FROM RECORDS

Patients often request information from their records. Written permission authorizing release of information should always be obtained and attached to the patient's record.

Patients sometimes ask for information to be sent to other doctors such as internists or neurologists. When patients move, they frequently want information transferred to an eye doctor located in their new vicinity. Copies of any reports or letters that were sent out should be maintained in the record. If any questions occur later as to why information was provided, or what information was sent, this will be available in the patient's record.

The general rule in releasing information is to provide the minimum amount of information to comply with the patient's request (Classe 1989a). Reports, summaries, or letters are usually sufficient to cover the necessary information. It is always better to find out what information the patient needs, than to provide the full record. Copies of the original should be provided only when absolutely necessary, such as in cases of litigation.

SPECTACLE AND CONTACT LENS PRESCRIPTIONS

The Federal Trade Commission's Eyeglass I rule granted patients a right to obtain information about spectacle and contact lens prescriptions. A fee can be charged for verifying spectacles or contact lenses acquired from other practitioners. If lenses are prescribed, a copy of the prescription, signed by the doctor, must be offered to the patient at the end of the examination. Minimum information on the prescription includes sphere, cylinder, axis, prism power, and prism orientation (when indicated). An expiration date can be written on the prescription, provided the date is reasonable.

Additional information, such as lens material, can be provided on the prescription. When safety glasses are intended, the doctor should write "polycarbonate lenses only" on the prescription, to limit liability if the lenses are purchased from another provider. Additional contact lens parameters for contact lens prescriptions are mandated by state regulations. For specific information on state laws, individual state regulating boards and the American Optometric Association can be contacted.

MAINTAINING RECORDS

When patient liability is concerned, it is important to remember that "out of sight is not out of mind." Even years after a patient has been seen, malpractice proceedings can be initiated. Statutes of limitations for malpractice— the period of time in which an individual can bring a claim against a doctor—vary from state to state. The duration of time in many state regulations is longer for minors, who can often file claims into adulthood.

It is important to retain records as useful evidence in the event of future claims. When can records be discarded? Ideally, it is said that records should never be discarded (Classe 1989a). Microfilm capabilities make it possible to preserve records without requiring excessive space. For doctors who choose to discard records at some point in time, the implications of the statutes of limitations, and possibilities for future liability, should be strongly considered.

CONFIDENTIALITY OF RECORDS

All members of the office staff must be aware of the confidentiality of information in a patient's record. Since there are often a number of people who handle records within an office, and staff members may have access to very personal information, it is important for all members of the office staff to be knowledgeable and respectful of patient confidentiality.

THE RECORD OF THE FUTURE

Records of the future may become computerized (Dister and Harris 1989; Ball and Collen 1992; Dick and Steen 1991). Although the paper-based record has been the basis of maintaining clinical information in the past, the introduction of the computerized clinical record raises some new issues. Computerized records permit doctors to have easy access to data, simply by calling up a patient's record. They also help solve the problem of illegibility. Opportunities for accessing data from different sites, if a doctor practices at different locations, are useful. Possibilities for transmitting data to a patient's other doctors may also become easier. It has been recommended that data acquisition for research purposes and insurance claims would be easier if records are stored electronically. It has also been suggested that a computer-stored clinical record would be the "ideal" context for automated decision support systems, since all of the information would already be entered in the computer (Ball and Collen 1992). Several issues, discussed below, are still complex.

DATA ENTRY

Investigators have found that doctors are eager to access patient data from the computer, but are less enthusiastic about entering information (Ball and Collen 1992). Several questions about data entry have been raised. Should results be handwritten and then entered into the computer? Should the doctor be responsible for entering the data into the computer, or should this be delegated to office staff? Can results be registered into the computer directly from instruments in the office? This complexity will probably be reduced as office computerization becomes increasingly simplified and adaptable in the future.

OPERATIONAL AND PROCEDURAL QUESTIONS

1. Most states require that a clinical record contain a doctor's written signature. How will the doctor *sign* the computer record? Individual access keys and passwords may enable doctors to confirm and identify their records.
2. When a new instrument or procedure is introduced in an office, an empty space on the paper record can be used for this purpose, until new records are printed. Paper records offer flexibility, since a note or comment can always be added to identify a new test.

   Adding new instruments and procedures necessitate alterations in the office computer program. Currently, many doctors would require the services of professional computer programmers to alter or modify the format for data input. This inconvenience will probably become less significant as more doctors and office staff members become familiar and comfortable with computer technology.
3. Paper-based records can accommodate external reports and data. Sheets and forms from external sources can be easily attached to a patient's paper record by taping, stapling, or clipping reports to the record. The mechanism for adding externally generated information into computerized records is still uncertain. Will accessory paper records be necessary to supplement computerized patient files?
4. Safeguards to protect data in the event of system failures will be necessary. Procedures to maintain adequate back-up files will be necessary to prevent accidental loss of information.

RECORD SECURITY AND PATIENT CONFIDENTIALITY

Computerized systems must provide security from unauthorized data access. In large health care institutions, many individuals have access to records. Multiple-user systems provide advantages in data retrieval, but inappropriate access must be prevented. Large computer systems are often linked to other institutional computers. Safeguards to protect clinical data and patient confidentiality will be needed. Individual access keys and passwords may assist in this task.

NOTE-TAKING DURING THE CASE HISTORY

Clinicians who take case histories frequently write information in the record as they interview the patient. Writing as the interviewer proceeds is helpful in recording the full information, without forgetting details. Recording the history from memory, at the end of the complete interview, would put the interviewer at a much greater risk of forgetting details.

Although recording as the case history proceeds has advantages, it is important to remember that note-taking can sometimes make the interviewer appear less attentive. Direct eye contact is a way of attending actively to a patient. When eye contact is interrupted a patient may feel that the doctor's attention is interrupted. The interviewer should be careful to maintain good listening skills while conducting the case history.

Recommendations discussed in Chapter 3 can help the interviewer maintain steady rapport with the patient, even while taking notes. It is especially important to remember to face a patient during the case history. Some interviewers like to lean on a counter that does not face the patient (Figure 9.2A), but this creates an obstacle to good communication. By maintaining an orientation in which the body is facing the patient (Figure 9.2B) the doctor is perceived as still attending to the patient, even with brief glances down at the record card. Clipboards held by the interviewer can serve the same purpose as a counter in providing a surface for writing.

Some doctors use case history forms that patients fill out themselves as they arrive for an examination. It is important to realize that although the doctor can obtain valuable information with these forms, many of the aspects of the interaction that usually occur during a traditional case history may be lost with this procedure. It is advisable to review at least the major parts of the history with patients, so patients know that the doctor is familiar with their concerns. Ignoring this step can greatly impede the doctor's ability to establish and build rapport with the patient.

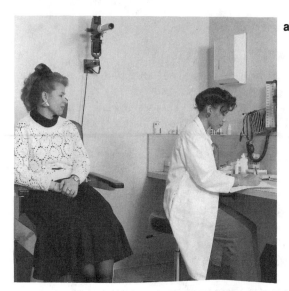

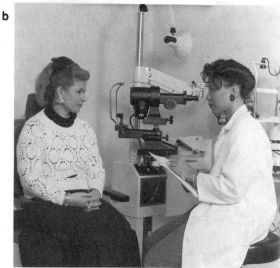

Figure 9.2 Taking notes during the interview. Doctors sometimes like to lean the record on a flat surface while taking notes, but when the counter or table is on the side this does not lead to good communication (a). It is important to face the patient and maintain good eye contact (b). Clipboards can be helpful for this purpose.

STRATEGIES FOR RECORDKEEPING

1. To improve your recordkeeping, remember the characteristics of good recordkeeping: comprehensive, well-organized, neat, legible records.
2. The Problem-Oriented Medical Record (POMR) can assist the doctor in improving the process and quality of recordkeeping. Using the four parts of the system (data base, problem list, plan list, and progress notes) can help the doctor maintain well-organized and logical records.
3. Clinical records have both short-term and long-term benefits. The doctor should take advantage of both aspects. Good records help the doctor on the day of the examination, and provide continuity in the future. Good records over time can improve continuity of care.
4. The clinician should be aware of legal issues that relate to recordkeeping. Office staff members should also be aware of these concepts. Good recordkeeping includes documentation of the case history, examination findings, patient management plans, and all patient communications. All recommendations for referrals and consultations should be recorded. Any telephone conversations with patients and consulting doctors should be recorded. Letters or reports from other doctors should be attached to the patient's record.
5. Clinical records should *never* be altered with the intention of covertly changing information. Altered records can result in serious consequences in the event of litigation, even if the practitioner performed all responsibilities adequately. When changes are necessary, the original entry should be crossed out with a single line. The doctor should sign or initial the new entry, and date it. A reason for the change should also be written. Once a record is called for litigation, changes should *never* be made to the record.
6. All canceled and missed appointments should be documented in the record. Attempts to contact the patient to reschedule, either by telephone or mail, should also be recorded. Document signs of noncompliance. These documentations can be valuable in the event of legal claims.
7. Contact lens cases comprise a large proportion of optometric malpractice cases. Informing patients about the potential risks and complications of contact lens wear is essential. Many doctors use preprinted forms to document patient education and informed consent.
8. Records of the future may utilize computer technology. Doctors should become familiar with the issues related to the introduction of computerized records.
9. Note-taking during the case history can interfere with eye contact. The doctor should take steps to maintain good eye contact and rapport with the patient during the clinical interview.

QUESTIONS FOR THOUGHT

1. What are the advantages and disadvantages of prelabeled record forms? blank sheets? What is your own preference for recordkeeping?
2. When you refer patients to another doctor, *what* information from your record do you transmit to the doctor? *How* do you convey the information about your records to the referred doctor (e.g., a Xeroxed copy of the actual record, a letter or report, a phone call)? Answer the above questions for the following situations:
   a. You are referring a diabetic patient to an ophthalmologist for a fluorescein angiogram.
   b. You have found increased hypertensive retinopathy, and you are referring a patient back to his general internist.
   c. A patient whom you have cared for over the last five years will be starting college in another state. The patient has asked that you contact an optometrist in that state with a record of the patient's clinical information.
3. How can you explain the risks and complications of contact lens wear to a patient without discouraging the patient from starting to wear lenses? Can long forms that require a patient's signature cause unnecessary panic and concern?
4. You happen to be going through some records and notice that you omitted an entry by mistake. You are looking at your records of an examination that took place three months ago. You performed a routine dilation on a patient. The drops that you used to dilate the patient are recorded appropriately, and most of the ophthalmoscopic findings are adequate; however, you notice that you forgot to fill in anything on your record about the periphery. You habitually write an entry on the record when you observe a retina that is flat and intact, with no holes or tears, but in this case you must have forgotten. You know that you always check, and you recall that you must have in this case, too. You reason to yourself: is three months too long to add an entry? Are you certain that your recall after three months is accurate? If the patient has a retinal detachment before the next examination, can you be held liable for missing a retinal hole or tear? What are your options for handling this situation and what would you do?
5. Are there any ways of predicting which patients are likely to become litigious? If an unsuccessful contact lens wearer suggests that legal claims may be initiated against you, how would you handle this situation?
6. You have cared for a patient for the past seven years, for both general eye care and contact lenses. The patient is moving to another city, and requests copies of her records. You offer to write a report to her new

doctor, but she adamantly insists on receiving Xeroxed copies of her record. How would you handle this situation?

7. How do you feel computerized recordkeeping would fit into your clinical environment? What are the advantages and disadvantages of automated recordkeeping? Is this the way of the future, or do you think that paper-based record systems will survive?

REFERENCES

Ball MJ, Collen MF. Aspects of the Computer-Based Patient Record. New York: Springer-Verlag, 1992.

Barresi BJ. Ocular Assessment. Boston: Butterworth-Heinemann, 1984.

Barresi BJ, Nyman NN. Implementation of the problem-oriented system in an optometric teaching clinic. American Journal of Optometry and Physiological Optics 55(11):765–770, 1978.

Classe JG. Legal Aspects of Optometry. Boston: Butterworth- Heinemann, 1989a.

Classe JG. A review of 50 malpractice claims. Journal of the American Optometric Association 60(9):694–706, 1989b.

Classe JG. Legal aspects of visual field assessment. Journal of the American Optometric Association 60(12):936–938, 1989c.

Classe JG, Alexander LJ. Clinical and legal issues in the management of patients with diabetes. Journal of the American Optometric Association 59(11):897–901, 1988.

Classe JG, Snyder C, Benjamin WJ. Documenting informed consent for patients wearing disposable lenses. Journal of the American Optometric Association 60(3):215–220, 1989.

Cormier LS, Cormier WH. Interviewing and Helping Skills for Health Professionals. Boston: Jones and Bartlett, 1986.

Dick RS, Steen EB. The Computer-Based Patient Record: An Essential Technology for Health Care. Washington, D.C.: National Academy Press, 1991.

Dister RE, Harris MG. Computerized optometric records and the law. Journal of the American Optometric Association 60(1):56–58, 1989.

Harris MG, Dister RE. Informed consent in contact lens practice. Journal of the American Optometric Association 58(3):230–236, 1987.

Kraushar MF. Recognizing and managing the litigious patient. Survey of Ophthalmology 37(1):54–56, 1992.

London R, Caloroso E, Barresi BJ. Problem orientation in vision therapy. American Journal of Optometry and Physiological Optics 58(5):393–399, 1981.

Scholles JR. Documentation and record keeping in clinical practice. Journal of the American Optometric Association 57(2):141–143, 1986.

Sloan PG. A "problem-oriented" optometric record? American Journal of Optometry and Physiological Optics 55(5):352–357, 1978.

Weed LL. Medical records that guide and teach. New England Journal of Medicine 278:593–600, 652–657, 1968.

Weed LL. Medical Records, Medical Education and Patient Care. Cleveland: Case Western Reserve, 1969.

ADDITIONAL READINGS

Bettman JW, Tennenhouse DJ. Some legal decisions significant for ophthalmology. Survey of Ophthalmology 32(1):32–34, 1987.

Hubler RS. Beyond the postcard. Optometric Economics 1(2):12–16, 1991.

Stamm J. Defensive optometry from the clinician's point of view. Prospectus 18(3):8–9, 1992.

Ziegler ML. Legal implications of optometric practice: Optometry from the attorney's point of view. Prospectus 18(4):7–8, 1992.

10

Interdisciplinary Interactions and Communications

Eye care problems are not isolated from other clinical problems. Since systemic problems have many ocular manifestations, optometrists can provide valuable clinical information to other health care professionals. Optometrists frequently interact with internists, neurologists, cardiologists, psychologists, occupational therapists, physical therapists, and other health care providers. Appropriate referrals and communication with other members of the health care delivery system can optimize the patient's overall clinical status. Improving the quality of interdisciplinary interactions can lead to improved clinical care.

Improved communications among the three Os—optometrist, ophthalmologist, and optician—can clearly improve the effectiveness of the eye care team and patient care. Recognizing each other's areas of expertise, and calling on each other's strengths, can optimize delivery of eye care services (Bennett 1987; Munson 1991; Soroka and Werner 1991; Bezan et al. 1992).

Interdisciplinary care is not limited just to health care professionals. Informing a teacher about a child's visual status and optometric intervention (e.g., new glasses, vision therapy) can help improve a patient's function and visual skills. Involving teachers, special educators, guidance counselors, and other educational personnel in the management of patients can result in enhanced compliance and improved clinical outcomes.

The health care worker in any specialty area, including eye care, does not operate within a vacuum that is separate and distinct from all other fields. Dr. Robert Rosenberg of the State University of New York–State College of Optometry reminds his students that "the patient is not just a pair of eyes." The patient is an individual with a unique combination of physical, social, and emotional factors that all may impact on a patient's function and health.

The patient's visual status and ocular health may affect, and be affected by, the patient's general medical status and overall clinical management. Ocular manifestations of systemic medical problems occur. Pharmacological agents used in the treatment of medical problems frequently have ocular side effects that need to be monitored. It is also possible for certain drugs used in the treatment of ocular problems to have various systemic side-effects. Each of these cases illustrates the importance of effective interdisciplinary relations.

Good interdisciplinary communications and cooperation can be instrumental in the overall management of a patient. Three types of interdisciplinary interactions will be discussed: consultation, referral, and comanagement. A model of interdisciplinary interactions and recommendations for effective teamwork will be presented in this chapter. Interprofessional collaboration is an example of the old "golden rule" that the whole is greater than the sum of its parts.

TYPES OF INTERDISCIPLINARY INTERACTIONS

Consultation

This type of clinical relationship occurs when a doctor sends a patient to another professional for (1) a specific test, (2) a set of tests, or (3) an expert opinion. The continuing care of the patient generally remains with the initial doctor, but the test results and opinions of the consulting doctor are helpful in identifying appropriate diagnoses and management plans. An example is an optometrist sending a patient with macular problems to an ophthalmologist for a fluorescein angiogram. The test results are helpful in enabling the doctor to choose appropriate management plans, and the patient is expected to return to the initial doctor for continuing care.

> A 49-year-old diabetic female is referred by her optometrist to an ophthalmologist for a fluorescein angiogram. The optometrist has identified an area of retinal exudates slightly temporal to the macula in one eye, and a possible area of macular edema.
>
> The optometrist telephones the ophthalmologist to provide information about the referral and to arrange a timely appointment for the patient. The optometrist describes what the test will entail to prepare the patient adequately. Prompt feedback from the ophthalmologist makes it possible to determine the appropriate management plan for the patient and the primary focus of continuing responsibility for care remains with the initial doctor.

Referral

Although referral and consultation are sometimes used interchangeably, referral generally indicates a transfer of responsibility that is expected to continue over an extended period of time. The patient may go back to the initial doctor after the problem is resolved, or the new doctor may be expected to take on long-term responsibility for managing the patient.

A 39-year-old male presents to his optometrist with symptoms of light flashes and floaters. The optometrist identifies a retinal detachment and refers the patient to a retinal specialist. The optometrist calls the ophthalmologist with information and the patient is seen the same afternoon. The optometrist explains to the patient that the ophthalmologist will handle the retinal surgery, but that after the retinal surgery and necessary follow-up, the patient will return to the optometrist for continuing ocular care in the future.

A 79-year-old male with macular degeneration has experienced a significant decrease in visual acuity. The optometrist notices that the patient is having extreme difficulty in adjusting to the reduced vision and in accepting the visual problem. He has also had some personal problems. The doctor recommends that the patient may find it helpful to discuss his concerns with a psychologist. The optometrist writes a letter to the local psychologist to explain the reason for the referral, and to provide relevant background information (Figure 10.1). In this case, the active care for the patient's mental health status is permanently transferred to the psychologist. Although the optometrist will continue to monitor the patient for his visual problems, the patient will see the psychologist for care related to his psychological status.

Comanagement

When a clinician brings in another health care provider with the intention of working *together* in caring for the patient, a comanagement relationship exists. In this relationship, both professionals are attending to the patient's problem, and both have some responsibility in monitoring the patient's status. In comanagement, responsibilities are shared; therefore, good communication and coordination of activities are imperative for successful interactions. An example is a patient with cataracts who is comanaged by an optometrist and an ophthalmologist. In many cases, the optometrist has served as the primary eye care provider for a period of time and is very familiar with the patient. The optometrist provides pre- and postsurgical care to his patient. The ophthalmologist performs care related to cataract surgery. In this relationship, the areas of expertise of both professionals are utilized and the patient benefits from the smooth interaction and collaboration.

A 68-year-old male presents to the optometrist with complaints of blurred vision in his right eye. Best corrected visual acuities are 20/70 in the right eye

Dr. Marlene Beck
52 Parker Street
New York, NY 10025

Dear Dr. Beck:

I am referring my patient, Philip Huddey, to you for a psychological evaluation. Mr. Huddey, a 79-year-old male, has had macular degeneration for the past 6 years. This condition has resulted in changes in the areas of his retina that are responsible for the clearest vision. He has experienced a significant reduction in his vision, especially in the past 6 months. Mr. Huddey's best corrected visual acuity at distance and near is 20/100 in the right eye, and 20/80 in the left eye.

I have noticed recently that Mr. Huddey seems unusually sad and reserved, unlike his normal personality. He appears to have lost a significant amount of weight, and he has also mentioned having problems falling asleep at night. He is having a difficult time adapting to some of the changes that have occurred in his life recently, and I have suggested that a psychological evaluation may be helpful.

I am continuing to monitor Mr. Huddey for his visual status. His next regular appointment with me will be in three months, but I have asked him to return right away if he notices any changes in his vision before then.

I hope this information is helpful. Please feel free to call me if I can be of any assistance.

Sincerely,

Elaine Jones

Elaine Jones, O.D.

Figure 10.1 Letter of referral to a psychologist.

and 20/30 in the left eye. The reduction in vision in both eyes is due to cataracts.

The optometrist chooses to refer the patient to an ophthalmologist with whom comanagement services for patients requiring cataract surgery are provided. In this type of arrangement, it is important for all individuals involved (the optometrist, the ophthalmologist, and the patient) to understand who will be responsible for various services. This type of interaction requires the greatest ongoing communication between professionals to prevent unnecessary repetition of tests, unintended omission of tests, and conflicting recommendations to the patient. In this case, the optometrist performs the presurgical evaluation; both doctors are involved to some extent in providing pre- and postoperative services. Eventually, the patient will be returned to the optometrist for future eye care, but for the period of time when cataract surgery is performed, both professionals share responsibility. A clear division and understanding of the activities, timing, and coordination of responsibilities are required by the optometrist and ophthalmologist for this arrangement to be successful.

EFFECTIVE COLLABORATION

In general, one form of collaboration is not necessarily preferable to the others, but a particular form may be better suited to certain types of problems. Depending on the types of services needed, and the health care professionals available, an appropriate form of interdisciplinary care should be selected by the initial doctor.

Of the three forms of collaboration, the comanagement arrangement requires the greatest level of ongoing communication during the care of the patient. The focus of responsibility of the patient also varies with the three types of interactions. In consultation, the ongoing responsibility for the patient is maintained by the initial doctor. In referral arrangements, the responsibility in monitoring and caring for a particular aspect of clinical care is usually transferred to a second doctor; in some cases, the initial doctor may maintain responsibility for other aspects of the patient's health care status. In the comanagement situation, both health care professionals are actively involved in monitoring and caring for the patient.

It should be noted that in the discussion on responsibility for the patient, the term "responsibility" is used to describe the focus of activity and management related to a patient's problem (or set of problems). Referral and consultation do not remove the initial doctor from legal responsibility. It therefore behooves the doctor to choose wisely in selecting referral and consultation sources, and in checking to make sure patients follow through with referral and consultation recommendations.

REFERRALS AND CONSULTATION ETIQUETTE

1. Doctors should provide the referral source or consultant with an adequate introduction and background on the patient, including a description of services needed. Telephone calls and written letters or reports (sent with the patient, or by mail) are all possibilities. The specific form of patient introduction and background should be decided on by the two doctors who are working together.

   One of the most difficult experiences for a consulting doctor is to have a patient show up in the office, and the reason for the consultation is unknown. The patient does not know why a referral was made, the referring doctor has not called or sent a letter, and the consultant does not know where to begin. Informing consultants of the reasons for referrals and consultations improves the quality of clinical care.

2. Make sure the expectations and respective responsibilities of the interprofessional interaction are made clear to all parties involved: the initial doctor, the second (consulting, referring, or comanaging) doctor, and the patient.

   A common obstacle to successful interactions occurs when the expectations of the individuals involved are not clear (Lipp 1986). Doctors sometimes say, "He stole my patient," or "Whenever I send a patient to that doctor, I never get that patient back." Unsatisfactory outcomes often occur when expectations are not clear.

If the patient is referred for a particular test, the doctor contacted should know that this is on a consulting basis. Patients should also be told the reason for the referral, the type of testing that will be performed, and directions for subsequent care. Sometimes it is difficult to predict the focus of future care until the test is performed.

In these cases, it is helpful to discuss the alternatives in advance, so the patient does not suddenly feel confused or surprised when the results are known and instructions are given to obtain further services. ("If everything is negative on the test, I'd like you to return to my office in a month so I can follow up; if there is a problem on the test, Dr. Trent will discuss some additional steps with you, depending on what is found.")

3. Prepare patients for tests and procedures that they will obtain from consulting doctors.

Patients are often nervous and anxious about going to a strange office, especially if they are worried about the potential outcomes and results. Doctors can help ease a patient's concern by explaining why a referral is necessary and what the tests entail. Understanding what will be done in the consulting doctor's office can also help the patient understand why some repetition of services may be necessary.

4. Reserve "emergency" referrals for situations that require an emergency basis.

Consultants are often inconvenienced by inappropriate "emergency" referrals. To maintain one's credibility with consulting doctors, it is important to preserve referrals that are made on an emergency basis for those cases that require timely intervention. When consulting doctors get a phone call from a doctor who has credibility, most will make immediate arrangements to see the patient.

5. Consulting doctors should remember that doctors who send patients to them expect their patients to be seen on a timely basis, and they expect timely feedback.

Feedback usually exists in the form of a written report. Written reports should be clear, concise, straightforward, neat, and respectful, thanking the initial doctors for their referrals and listing their proper titles (e.g., not Ms. or Mr. when it should be Dr.). Lengthy, verbose reports make it harder for the doctor to glean useful, relevant information.

It is also important to use language appropriately. Doctors tend to use a lot of complicated terms and jargon that are not shared by professionals in other specialty areas. If not adequately explained, convergence problems to the eye care doctor may be confused with convergent problems to the psychologist or psychiatrist. When collaborating with other health care professionals, it is important to define one's terms to the other health care provider, as necessary, and to be conscious of the way in which language is used differently between professions.

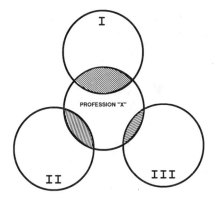

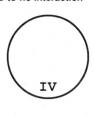

Level I: Frequent Collaboration and Interaction
Level II: Moderate Collaboration and Interaction
Level III: Limited Collaboration and Interaction
Level IV: Rare-to-no Interaction

Figure 10.2 Model of interdisciplinary interactions. Interprofessional collaboration can be demonstrated by a central circle (Profession "X") and overlapping circles. Level I: Frequent collaboration and interaction. Health care workers in this category frequently work with Profession "X." Level II: Moderate collaboration and interaction. Health care workers in this category sometimes come into contact with Profession "X" but less frequently or intensely than with those in Level I. Level III: Limited collaboration and interaction. Health care workers in this category interact less frequently with Profession "X" than those in Levels I and II, but when they do interact, cooperation is essential. Level IV: Rare-to-no interaction. Health care workers in this category have minimal to no contact and interaction with Profession "X." Although the importance of these areas is recognized, they do not frequently interact or work together in the care of patients.

6. Doctors involved in collaborative arrangements should be conscious of the importance of treating each other respectfully.

    Referrals and consulting professionals are selected by areas of expertise. The confident consultant makes the referring doctor look good in front of patients for making appropriate referrals. When questions about referrals arise, these should be discussed directly with the initial doctor.

    In all verbal and written interactions, collaborating doctors should be sensitive to the recommendations of "referral etiquette" that can make interdisciplinary care more effective.

MODEL OF INTERDISCIPLINARY INTERACTION

A model of interdisciplinary interaction and collaboration can be applied to specific health professions and their interactions with other health care providers (Figure 10.2). The profession discussed (Profession "X") and its responsibilities and activities are represented by the central circle.

Figure 10.2 demonstrates levels of interaction. In Level I, the area of overlap of the circles is greater than the areas for Levels II, III, and IV, demonstrating more frequent interaction and collaboration. Level IV is

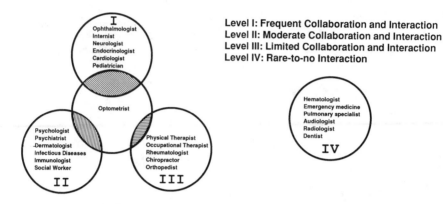

Level I: Frequent Collaboration and Interaction
Level II: Moderate Collaboration and Interaction
Level III: Limited Collaboration and Interaction
Level IV: Rare-to-no Interaction

Figure 10.3 Optometric collaboration. An example of an optometrist's interprofessional relationships. Other optometrists may have different profiles, and an optometrist's profile may change over time. For an explanation of Levels I–IV see the legend to Figure 10.2.

totally distinct from the circle of Profession "X," indicating the absence of collaboration. (The separation and differentiation do not suggest a lack of regard for the area of the other discipline, only a reflection that the two professions do not frequently interact.)

Several points should be made about this model:

1. Different professionals have different profiles. Figure 10.3 shows an example of an optometrist's relationship with other health care providers.
2. Individuals within the same profession who practice in different types of environments may draw their profiles differently. An optometrist who works with a lot of children may include pediatricians in Level I or II; one who sees few children may list pediatricians in Level IV. An optometrist who works in a private practice may have a different profile from one who works in a hospital-based setting.
3. An individual professional's profile may change over time, as the demographics of his or her patient population changes, and as other professionals in the same local area change.
4. The profile helps illustrate the possibilities for collaboration and interaction with other professionals. The model also helps to demonstrate that health care providers should also consider the possibilities for interaction within their own profession (e.g., within the same central circle). This is most apt to occur when health care professionals do not choose to provide all of the services that are potentially provided by individuals within their profession. For example, optometrists may

choose to refer some of their patients to other optometrists specializing in low vision, contact lenses, or vision therapy, if they do not provide these services.

Several characteristics of relationships within this model can be considered in studying one's interactions with other health care providers:

1. *Areas of overlapping responsibilities:* Overlapping responsibilities occur most frequently with Level I providers. Optometrists and ophthalmologists both carry out some of the same functions, so a clear understanding of expectations and responsibilities of both professionals is important for smooth interaction. When overlapping responsibilities exist, and clinical management of patients is not well coordinated, unnecessary repetition and accidental omission of tests can occur. Expectations should be clearly outlined in these interactions and doctors should avoid making assumptions. When in doubt, it is better to contact the other doctor, or to repeat the test so crucial information is not overlooked. Good communication between interacting doctors would eliminate these types of potential confusions.
2. *Areas of true collaboration:* These are opportunities for clinical care in which both professionals can work together in a patient's best interests. The comanagement arrangement, described previously, is an example of a relationship exemplified by true collaboration. In activities such as the management of a patient for cataract surgery, the active participation and expertise of both professionals can benefit the patient.
3. *Areas of possible conflict:* When health care providers are involved in the management of similar problems, and they have different perspectives and philosophies in patient management, potential conflicts may arise. Patients with the same problem may be advised differently by the two health professionals, and this can be confusing to the patient. Many optometrists and ophthalmologists handle decisions on vision therapy differently. Similarly, surgeons and nonsurgical medical specialists sometimes advise patients differently on their opinions for, or against, surgery. Health care professionals should be aware of areas of potential conflict in their fields and the effect that the conflict can have on patients.

The relationships illustrated in this model can be improved with the use of referral/consultation etiquette. By being aware of the areas of overlapping responsibilities, true collaboration, and possible conflict, health care professionals can improve interdisciplinary communication and the quality of patient care.

OBSTACLES TO GOOD INTERDISCIPLINARY INTERACTIONS

Improving clinical care requires the management of potential obstacles to communication. Figure 1.3 illustrates basic obstacles to good communication. A special set of obstacles that play a significant role in interfering with effective communications with other clinicians is presented:

1. *Egos:* If health care professionals believe that their area of expertise is more important to the patient than another, egos can get in the way of effective interdisciplinary interactions.
2. *Biases and viewpoints:* If health care providers hold different viewpoints and perspectives on patient management, areas of potential conflict and confusion can occur.
3. *"Turf" issues:* When specialties share potential areas of overlap, professionals are sometimes concerned about maintaining their responsibility. They may worry about others encroaching on their territory. These concerns of "turf" and "territoriality" often prevent effective interprofessional collaboration.
4. *History of interprofessional relations:* When professions have a history of pressured relationships, often resulting from long-standing political concerns, individual practitioners frequently carry on and perpetuate these feelings. It can sometimes take a long time to "undo" many years of strained relations. In the interest of optimal patient care, health professionals can work to improve communications and interactions between different clinical specialty areas.

EFFECTIVE TEAMWORK

Eye care professionals frequently have occasion to serve as members of a team. Some optometrists work on teams evaluating children with perceptual and learning disabilities. Others work as part of rehabilitative teams for patients who have experienced head trauma and strokes. In these cases, the interaction of the professionals involved is central to the success of the team.

As a member of the team, the optometrist's role involves diagnosis, management, and information exchange (Zambone 1990). Responsibility no longer stops at identifying an optometric management plan. Sharing evaluations and assessments is an integral part of the team member's interaction.

The doctor working as part of a team should be aware of five stages in handling cases: background, examination and evaluation, information exchange, integration, and outcome (Figure 10.4).

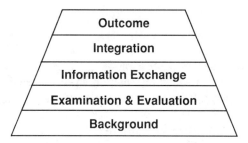

Figure 10.4 Effective teamwork. Effective teamwork can be characterized by five stages: background, examination and evaluation, information exchange, integration, and outcome.

Background

Made up of two components, the background of the case involves the combined backgrounds of the team and the patient. Each team should have a statement of purpose that concisely explains the functions and goals of that team. This can help members understand how each contributes to the group. The other is the background of the patient who presents to the team. The patient's specific background can be established through the case history and any introductory materials supplied to the doctor by the team coordinator. It is important to understand the patient's unique situation to make meaningful decisions.

Examination and Evaluation

Clinical testing, assessment, and diagnosis are primary functions of the health care professional who functions as part of a team.

Information Exchange

Having made an evaluation, the doctor's impressions must be communicated to the other members of the team. There is usually an agreed on procedure for this. The eye doctor may send a written report, provide input over the telephone, or both. It is important for the process of information exchange to be acceptable to all the members of the team. The eye care professional may also attend multidisciplinary conferences on patients.

Integration

Once the individual components of the evaluation have been carried out, information from different professionals must be put together to produce the outcome. There is usually one person who is responsible for the integration of information. The optometrist should be familiar with the team coordinator, and with how the coordinator collects and integrates information. Once the information is submitted to the team coordinator, team members should make themselves available for follow-up questions.

Outcome

The teamwork leads to a desired outcome: an educational placement for a child, a clinical diagnosis or classification for a patient, or a rehabilitation plan. These are just a few examples, but teams may work toward various outcomes. It is important for the optometrist to be aware of the type of outcome that is sought at the outset of each case, so relevant tests are done, and appropriate information is provided to the team coordinator.

Optometrists may be asked to provide a variety of services as part of an interdisciplinary team, including general optometric services, vision therapy evaluations and programs, perceptual work-ups and therapy, low vision care, and vision rehabilitation services. Recommendations on academic placement, educational goals, classroom seating, vocational placement, and environmental factors (e.g., proper lighting, placement of books) may also be sought. Eye care professionals can provide valuable insights that can improve a patient's ability to function within their school, work, and vocational programs.

An 8-year-old boy with cerebral palsy is evaluated by an optometrist as part of the multidisciplinary team. The teachers are requesting information about the ability of this patient to see and use his vision, since they have had limited success in getting him to look at books and other detailed targets.

The optometrist finds that this patient is a high hyperope, with a constant left esotropia (40Δ). The patient has an old pair of glasses that needs to be changed. Even with the new prescription, the patient's visual acuity is assessed as poor in both eyes, with the vision in the left eye worse as a result of amblyopia. The doctor also finds that the patient has a left lateral gaze palsy in both eyes. This means that the patient's ability to move his eyes to his left is limited. By informing the teachers who work with the patient about this finding, and its implications, the optometrist can improve the effectiveness of the educator's hard work and efforts. The doctor recommends that visual targets be presented either straight ahead or to the patient's right. Presenting food, or visual targets, from the patient's left can result in frustration and reduced responses. The doctor also recommends that books and targets with large letters be used because of the patient's visual acuity. Using the doctor's recommendations, the teachers are now able to get the patient to recognize letters and pictures. They also observe that the child is more responsive visually since they have become aware of the direction from which they present visual targets. At a multidisciplinary conference, it is observed that this patient is now able to function at a higher level in his activities.

STRATEGIES FOR IMPROVING INTERDISCIPLINARY COMMUNICATIONS

Improved interdisciplinary interactions should allow for efficient utilization of all health care professionals and optimal communication.

1. Be aware of the three forms of interdisciplinary collaboration: consultation, referral, and comanagement.
2. Understand the characteristics of "referral etiquette," and be conscious of adhering to these recommendations when interacting with other professionals (see pp. 141–143).
3. Consider the other professionals with whom you interact, and the levels at which these interactions occur (e.g., Level I, Level II, Level III, Level IV).
4. Be conscious of areas of overlap, of true collaboration, and of potential conflict. Be aware of possible obstacles that can impede good interprofessional interactions. Good communications between the professionals involved can eliminate many potential problems and optimize interdisciplinary relationships.
5. Remember the five stages of handling cases as a team member: background, examination and evaluation, information exchange, integration, and outcome. Effective teamwork requires appropriate interdisciplinary collaboration.

QUESTIONS FOR THOUGHT

1. The lists of interacting professionals in Figure 10.5 have been left blank. Consider the professionals with whom you interact. Draw your profile by writing providers in the circles, at the appropriate levels. (Use Figure 10.3 as an example.) If you are a student, write in the profile for the type of environment in which you intend to practice.
2. You receive a letter from another doctor that you feel is unclear. The letter is lengthy and contains a lot of information, but it includes terms with which you are not familiar. What do you do about this?
   a. Do you contact the doctor to discuss this situation, or should you use the information that is provided as well as possible?
   b. Would you work with this health professional again?

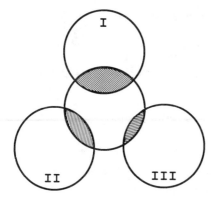

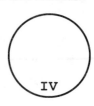

Level I: Frequent Collaboration and Interaction
Level II: Moderate Collaboration and Interaction
Level III: Limited Collaboration and Interaction
Level IV: Rare-to-no Interaction

Figure 10.5 Design your own model of interdisciplinary interactions. For an explanation of Levels I–IV see the legend to Figure 10.2.

3. Your staff member informs you that a consulting doctor is on the telephone and would like to speak to you. The doctor is calling to discuss a patient whom you have referred on a nonemergency basis, and you do not anticipate that there is any serious problem. You want to be polite and speak with the doctor, but you are in the middle of an examination and your reception room is full of patients waiting for you. Do you take the call? Do you tell your staff person that you will return the call? Do you ask the staff person to take the information for you? How would you handle this situation?

4. Discuss six recommendations for effective referrals and consultations. How do you apply these recommendations in your clinical setting?

5. You referred a patient to another health care provider. The patient informs you that the other doctor provided conflicting information and that the other doctor said that your recommendations are "wrong." What do you say to the patient? How would you handle this situation?

6. Select a patient that you have examined recently and review the patient's clinical findings.
   a. Write a letter that would be appropriate to send to the patient's general internist.
   b. Write a letter that would be appropriate for the patient's teacher.
   c. Write a letter that would be appropriate for the patient's psychologist.
   d. Write a letter for a specialist caring for a particular clinical problem of the patient (e.g., a cardiologist, neurologist, endocrinologist).
   How would these letters be different? How would they be similar?

REFERENCES

Bezan D, Halverson K, Schaffer K, Thomas P. Optometric Guide to Surgical Co-management. Boston: Butterworth-Heinemann, 1992.

Bennett I. The three O's in perspective. Optometric Management 22:44–47, 1987.

Lipp MR. Respectful Treatment—A Practical Handbook of Patient Care. New York: Elsevier Science Publishing, 1986.

Munson BJ. Doctor to doctor—Building better referral relationships with ophthalmologists. Optometric Economics 1(9):35–38, 1991.

Soroka J, Werner DL. Optometry and ophthalmology: Renewed professional rivalry. Journal of the American Optometric Association 62:283–287, 1991.

Zambone A. Optometrists on the team: Holistic care and the patient–parent–educator interface. In Rosenbloom AA, Morgan MW, eds., Principles and Practice of Pediatric Optometry. Philadelphia: J.B. Lippincott, 1990: 560–576.

ADDITIONAL READINGS

Hellerstein LF, Fishman B. Vision therapy and occupational therapy. Journal of Behavioral Optometry 1:122–126, 1990.

Hubler RS. Confident, competent referrals. Optometric Economics 2(8):14–17, 1992.

Kalb L, Warshowsky JH. Occupational therapy and optometry: Principles of diagnosis and collaborative treatment of learning disabilities in children. Occupational Therapy Practice 3:77–87, 1991.

Muzzin LJ. Understanding the process of medical referral—Parts 1–6. Canadian Family Physician 37:2155–2161, 1991; 38:532–538, 1992.

World Health Organization. Learning to work together for health. Geneva: World Health Organization Technical Report Series 769, 1988.

11

Doctor–Staff Communications

For many patients, the first contact with the office is through members of the office staff. Before they ever meet the doctor, patients usually call for an appointment. As they arrive at the office, they are greeted by a member of the staff. When patients call the office, what impression do they receive? Do they hear a pleasant, friendly voice? When they arrive for their appointment, what attitude do they sense? Do they feel a warm, supportive atmosphere, or a rushed, impersonal air?

The "office attitude" is, to a great extent, a product of the tone set by the whole team. The doctor is not the only individual who makes a strong impression on the patient. Every member of the office staff—from the person who answers the phones, to the one who greets the patients, to the one who handles billing—contributes to the quality of the clinical encounter.

It is estimated that 75% of mistakes made in the workplace can be attributed to ineffective communication, and that 80% of business losses occur because an employee communicates an attitude of indifference (Pryor 1987). For further discussion on communication skills for managers refer to Clampitt (1991), Drury (1984), Blanchard and Lorber (1984), and Blanchard and Johnson (1982); for health care professionals refer to Miller (1990), Leebov et al. (1990), and Aluise (1987). Better communications between the doctor and staff members can contribute significantly to the success of the practice.

Knowing how to supervise, delegate, provide feedback, and motivate workers does not automatically occur with the development of good clinical skills. Hunsaker and Alessandra (1980) point out that no matter how much expertise and technical skill you have, you cannot be an effective manager without knowing how to establish and maintain productive relationships with other individuals.

Good doctor–staff communications can make the office more effective: workers are more productive and better satisfied with their activities. A clear understanding of the roles and responsibilities of each member of the team is a primary requirement for an office that runs smoothly and harmoniously. Office flow, telephone communications, and staff training must all be handled effectively. Hiring new staff is one of the special challenges of doctor–staff communications and recommendations and strategies on interviewing will be discussed in this chapter. The outcome is an improved clinical environment for patients, and for the quality of their care.

OFFICE FLOW

For the office to run smoothly, all members of the office have to have a clear idea of their roles and responsibilities and how their tasks interact with the other activities and members in the office.

If members of the staff are unclear about their own responsibilities and about how their jobs relate to other work in the office, the result can be confusion and lost efficiency. If they are unsure of office policies, they may not conform to the doctor's priorities; this may be, however, because they are not aware of the doctor's unwritten or unspoken "rules."

Many doctors provide written manuals outlining the policies and procedures of the office (Wood 1992). The manuals may include information such as the philosophy of the practice, job descriptions, information on performance evaluations, work hours, employee benefits, sick leave, and vacation time. Information about appointment scheduling, fees, billing procedures, telephone responsibilities, confidentiality of records, and specific instructions on patient management may also be included. Many doctors also include copies of office forms and patient education handouts.

Office procedure manuals are very useful in clarifying the goals and flow of the office. They are especially helpful to new employees who are not sure of certain procedures; continuing employees can also refer to the manual when questions arise. It is important to update office manuals periodically, as jobs and responsibilities change or as procedures are modified.

Each individual must be competent in his or her responsibilities, but doctors and staff members must also work well together so their tasks and activities are well coordinated. The interactions of doctor and staff, and staff members with other members of the team, are instrumental in the resulting flow and administration of practice activities.

THE OFFICE ATTITUDE

How does the patient feel when arriving at the office? Comfortable and at ease? Apprehensive and nervous? The tone of the office is projected by all of the members of the office team. No single member of the team is more important than any other member in the overall success and satisfaction of the patient visit. Each person contributes to the quality of the clinical encounter.

Seven qualities of doctor–patient rapport were examined earlier: respect, concern, understanding, trust, empathy, sensitivity, and sincerity. Staff members should be aware of and demonstrate each of these qualities (see Chapter 6). Their effectiveness in projecting these qualities contributes to the office attitude. Ultimately, each member of the staff contributes to the caring message conveyed by the practice. All members who interact with patients can build therapeutic, helping interactions.

TELEPHONE COMMUNICATIONS

Telephone communications can usually be divided into three types of calls: appointments, inquiries, and emergencies.

Appointments

When patients call to make an appointment, their first impression is affected by the "office attitude." If the individual answering the phone sounds caring and concerned, this can create a favorable impression.

It has been said that the caller can "hear" a smile; it is recommended that staff members smile when they answer the phone. A pleasant voice and a warm, polite manner can create a positive introduction to the practice.

Many offices find it helpful to have appointment scripts. When patients call for appointments, or when assistants call patients to make appointments, these outlines ensure that all of the appropriate information is gathered. Scripts are particularly helpful when staff members call patients to schedule or reschedule appointments, since they provide potential responses for patients who express resistance toward making the appointment. Appointment scripts frequently include aspects of patient education. An assistant calling a patient suspected of having glaucoma to reschedule a missed appointment may tell the patient that the doctor is concerned because glaucoma can proceed without any symptoms, and without treatment it can cause significant visual loss. With preprogrammed office scripts, the office assistant is prepared for common situations that may occur.

Inquiries

Patients often call to ask about services provided in the office. "Does Dr. Jones fit contact lenses?" or "Does Dr. Robinson do vision therapy?" It is especially helpful to be able to inform old patients of new services that are provided in the office.

Some of the more difficult phone calls are from "telephone shoppers." Individuals frequently call around checking for prices. The strategy in handling these phone calls is to impress the caller with the quality of services that is provided.

Responding with a fee alone does little to describe the care. Before the actual fee is stated, it is often effective to stress the extent of the services. Comparing fees across offices does not provide a comparison of services. "Our fee for a general examination, which includes an eye health examination, determination of your prescription, evaluation of your focusing skills, assessment of color vision, and a glaucoma test, is fifty-five dollars." This can be much more effective than simply saying "fifty-five dollars." Sometimes it is not possible to give an exact fee because the assistant does not know what the patient needs. In quoting a fee, the assistant may be able to give a range: "The fee for our contact lenses is $125 to $425, depending on the type of lens."

It is usually helpful to engage the patient in some questions to demonstrate the quality of service provided in the office. "Are you interested in soft contact lenses or rigid lenses, Ms. Whitman? Are you thinking about getting daily wear lenses or extended wear?" It is also helpful to provide some patient education. "The doctor has to examine you to decide exactly what type of lens is best for you. That depends on the curvature of your cornea, your prescription, and your eye health." By this point, the patient may become very confident and comfortable with the office, and an appointment can be scheduled. In many cases, the exact fee that the patient hears is probably less important than the level of warmth and support sensed. In fact, "telephone shoppers" often schedule with offices that have higher fees when they become impressed with the quality and support of the care provided. The initial goal at this point is to gain the patient's trust.

Discussing fees successfully is especially important when a "consumerist" doctor–patient interaction is suggested by the patient (see Chapter 6).

Emergencies

Office staff must be well trained in how to handle telephone emergencies. Since staff members make appointments, they actually hold considerable responsibility for certain decisions. Under what circumstances should they tell a patient to come in to the office immediately? When is it acceptable to wait a few days, or a week? Office staff members should be reminded never to answer questions or to offer advice beyond their level of responsibility. When there is a question, or they are not sure of an answer, they should always consult with the doctor. Instruct staff on appropriate handling of emergencies. Different offices may have different procedures, but it is important for each office to have a well-planned, well-coordinated method for handling emergency situations including:

Chemical burns and chemical contact with the eye (e.g., lye, ammonia, acid solutions)

Flashes of light

Sudden acute loss of vision or loss of visual field (e.g., curtains, veils, blackouts)

Ocular injury and trauma

Foreign bodies and ocular pain

Postoperative patients with pain, redness, or reduced vision

The occurrence of chemical burns is a special category because it requires immediate action. Patients should be told to irrigate the eye immediately, and to continue irrigating. Asking the patient to leave home or work to come in for an appointment immediately would waste valuable initial time. The most important action in this situation is to start and maintain irrigation. When a phone call of this nature occurs, the doctor should be informed by the office staff immediately to ensure appropriate follow-up.

DOCTOR–STAFF INTERACTIONS

The doctor can support the philosophy and enthusiasm transmitted by the paraoptometric with frequent communication. Regular staff meetings provide valuable forums for discussions and provide the team with an opportunity to review problems that have occurred. Since staff members handle many of the daily occurrences, they are often in a position to identify the most helpful solutions. In addition, when staff members are involved in the process, they may be more likely to be supportive of the resulting decisions.

Aside from being a clinician, the doctor is a leader. The doctor must be able to supervise, delegate, provide feedback, and motivate the staff.

Effective Supervision

Effective supervision and delegation involves being specific, clear, timely, assertive, respectful, and sensitive. When responsibilities are delegated, tasks should be specific and clear. Expectations of the paraoptometric should be clearly defined. Feedback should be specific and timely, and performance evaluations should be provided regularly. Sensitivity to members of the office staff is a primary factor in building effective teamwork.

Effective Staff Training

Training members of the staff is largely an effort of communications. Again, specific, clear, and timely instructions are helpful. When office staff are taught to handle new procedures, or new staff members are hired, effective training is essential. Without good training, office workers may not perform their activities properly, and the doctor may question the worker's ability to perform.

A five-step guide to teaching office staff, adapted from Blanchard and Lorber (1984), and applied to the clinical environment, is provided:

1. Tell the learner what to do (verbal).
2. Show the learner how to do it (visual and tactual).
3. Encourage the learner to ask questions.
4. Let the learner try and practice.
5. Provide feedback and guidance.

The use of various senses (e.g., visual, auditory, kinesthetic) in patient teaching discussed in Chapter 8 is also pertinent to staff teaching. As the learner improves, less guidance and feedback may be needed.

Effective Feedback

Feedback to employees should be timely, specific, constructive, and supportive. Immediate feedback encourages staff members to remember exactly what they did or did not do. When feedback is specific, it is easier to make corrective steps. Constructive feedback should be presented in a way that allows the staff member to make positive changes. When it is supportive, it is easier for the individual to accept and utilize comments.

Communications experts often recommend using "I" language (Drury 1984). With "I" statements, speakers express their views about the other person's actions, but it does not come across as a personal attack on the individual. "You" messages tend to create defensiveness. Consider the two examples, below:

"I" language:
"I feel that it is a problem when you arrive at work late."
"I feel that you're not listening when I speak to you."

"You" language:
"You always come to work late."
"You never listen to me."

In both "I" statements, the speaker focuses on the behavior. In the "you" statements, the speaker appears to criticize the individual, and not the behavior. Communication experts (Meiss 1990) say to "focus on the performance, not the performer." In these situations, you are trying to change the action, not necessarily the person. Feedback is more effective when it addresses the specific behavior.

Feedback should also be expressed in positive terms, so the worker can make a change. Tell the worker what you want not what you do not want done. Say

I feel that it is more effective to answer the telephone in a friendly, helpful tone.

rather than

Don't sound so hurried and impolite each time you answer the telephone.

It is also recommended that office managers not limit performance comments to negative feedback. Managers should congratulate and acknowledge workers when they do something right. Workers often feel that they are taken for granted when they perform adequately; very often, they receive feedback only when they do something wrong. Providing positive feedback is an important aspect of training, and it can go a long way in building staff motivation and morale.

Motivating Staff

Building motivation and effective teamwork is an important responsibility of the leader. Workers tend to be most productive and loyal to an office if they are made to feel that they are valuable members of the team. One of the best sources of motivation is the leader. The leader should be a positive role model, demonstrating professionalism and warmth consistently. The level of enthusiasm and commitment of the leader to the patients in the practice can serve as a source of inspiration to the other members of the team.

Providing positive recognition and feedback is an easy way to motivate and encourage. Effective training and sensitive feedback can be helpful in allowing workers to develop to their highest potential. As they gain experience and expertise, workers are often interested in gaining higher levels of responsibility. When this is consistent with the needs of the practice, all members of the team—the doctor, staff, and patients—can benefit. Staff training and development are effective methods of motivating employees. Enhanced knowledge leads to improved self-esteem, confidence, and effectiveness. The rewards of staff training cycle directly back to the practice.

Doctors and office managers can build motivation by setting, and expressing, high expectations. When expressed supportively and enthusiastically, these expectations can provide motivation for optimal performance.

HIRING NEW EMPLOYEES

One of the most difficult aspects of running a practice is hiring the appropriate individuals. The members of the team determine how effectively the office will run and function. An initial step in hiring new employees is the interview.

Appendix C provides a list of questions for interviewing the potential office assistant. Ultimately, the interview should be more conversational than constant rapid-fire questioning. A set of questions prepared in advance can help the interviewer conduct the meeting. Understanding the applicant's employment history, goals, personal effectiveness, and interest in the particular job can provide insights into the applicant's suitability for the position.

The doctor may also want to ask the applicant specific questions that relate to the clinical environment. The following are examples of the types of questions that can be posed:

How would you handle a patient who complains because you are not able to schedule an appointment when the patient wants one?

How would you handle a patient who is angry because the patient is not seen by the doctor on time?

How would you handle a patient who appears to be very nervous when waiting to see the doctor?

These questions can help provide insights into an individual's interpersonal skills and effectiveness.

Once an individual is hired, the doctor should be conscious of the new employee's entry into the practice. New workers should have a clear understanding of the office flow and how their responsibilities and tasks interact with those of other office members. When job responsibilities and interactions are not clearly defined, misconceptions can occur and can often interfere with effective relationships between staff members.

It is especially important for new staff members to become familiar with professional terminology that is used in the office (Miller 1990). Workers should also be conscious of the recordkeeping aspects of their jobs, and the need to maintain clear, legible records so other people in the office can read their entries.

In addition to helping the new staff member fit into the practice, it is often helpful to team the member up with an employee who can serve as a positive role model in both function and attitude. An exemplary staff member can serve as a positive role model by demonstrating a high performance level and an enthusiastic commitment to the patients in the practice.

STRATEGIES FOR DOCTOR–STAFF COMMUNICATIONS

The effectiveness of doctor–staff communications contributes significantly to the success of the practice. The following recommendations can help the doctor create a more positive environment for all members of the team: the doctor, staff members, and patients.

1. All office members should be familiar with the division of responsibilities and the flow of the office. Misunderstandings can create disharmony. Clear roles and job descriptions are essential for smooth practice management.
2. The doctor should be conscious of the "office attitude" that is projected by the team. Every member of the office can create an impression on the patient. A comfortable, secure clinical environment depends on the commitment of all members of the team.
3. All workers in the office should be conscious of how they demonstrate the seven qualities of positive patient interaction: respect, concern, understanding, trust, empathy, sensitivity, and sincerity.
4. Members of the office staff should be trained in telephone communications. Encourage staff to smile when answering the phone. It has been said that callers can "hear" a smile at the end of the phone.
5. All staff members who answer the telephone should be trained in handling telephone emergencies. They should be familiar with the list of emergencies, and they should know how to handle patients who call in with these problems.
6. Doctors who run practices should master the aspects of effective supervision. Providing training, feedback, and motivation are essential functions in leading a successful team. There are many books devoted to these topics at local libraries and book stores. Some of them are listed at the end of this chapter, but there are also many other good ones that are available.
7. Use the five-step model to train staff members (see p. 157).
8. Expectations of staff should be clearly defined. Feedback is most effective when it is timely, specific, constructive, and supportive. Provide feedback regularly and remember to use "I" language to address behaviors; "you" language is confrontational and attacks the individual.
9. Managers are usually conscious of providing negative feedback, but they should also make sure that they provide positive feedback. Recognize the strengths of individuals, and they become stronger.

10. Hiring new employees is a challenging aspect of practice management. Look for employees who are capable, enthusiastic, and committed. A list of questions (Appendix C) can be helpful in guiding the interview.
11. When new workers start at the office, facilitate their entry by orienting them to the office flow. New workers should be introduced to the others in the office to develop effective relationships among staff members.
12. Good managers must be effective at motivating staff.

Doctors who run clinical practices should also remember the following:

1. Make each staff member feel like a valuable member of the team. (Each worker is a valuable member.)
2. Provide positive recognition for good work.
3. Hold high expectations for workers.
4. Provide staff training to enhance knowledge, performance, and self-esteem.
5. Serve as a positive role model. The doctor's energy, commitment, and professionalism can create an enthusiastic atmosphere.

QUESTIONS FOR THOUGHT

1. Write an outline for an office procedures manual. Include all of the topics that you feel are important to address in a manual. Which of the components are likely to change over time? Which are likely to be stable? How often do you anticipate you would need to update your manual?
2. The office flow and attitude make an important impression on the patient. Assume that you have just hired a new employee. How would you express your thoughts on the office attitude to the new assistant? What steps can you take to educate her about the office flow?
3. Write an "office script" for an office assistant who will be calling several patients with glaucoma who have not returned to your office for their follow-up visits. Be sure to include all possible comments of resistance by patients, and appropriate responses for your office assistant.
4. You want to train a new office staff member to insert and remove contact lenses. Describe your training program for this employee.
5. Discuss three methods of motivating members of your office staff.
6. You are planning to hire a new office assistant. You have been interviewing candidates, and have narrowed it down to two choices. One individual has more experience in the tasks that will be performed, but you are not sure about the level of this individual's interpersonal effectiveness.

The other candidate is warm and outgoing, but would require more training. Which one would you choose? Why?

7. You want to provide feedback to a staff member who consistently arrives at the office late in the morning and after lunch. With the exception of these actions, the performance of this staff member is excellent. How would you discuss this with your employee?

REFERENCES

Aluise JJ. The Physician as Manager. New York: Springer-Verlag, 1987.

Blanchard K, Johnson S. The One Minute Manager. New York: Berkley Books, 1982.

Blanchard K, Lorber R. Putting the One Minute Manager to Work. New York: Berkley Books, 1984.

Clampitt PG. Communicating for Managerial Effectiveness. Newbury Park, CA: Sage Publications, 1991.

Drury SD. Assertive Supervision—Building Involved Teamwork. Champaign, IL: Research Press, 1984.

Hunsaker P, Alessandra AJ. The Art of Managing People. New York: Simon & Schuster, 1980.

Leebov W, Vergare M, Scott G. Patient Satisfaction—A Guide to Practice Enhancement. Oradell, NJ: Medical Economics Books, 1990.

Meiss R. How to Listen Powerfully. Boulder, CO: CareerTrack Publications, 1990.

Miller P. The Vision Care Assistant—An Introductory Handbook. Santa Ana, CA: VisionExtension, 1990.

Pryor F. The Energetic Manager. Englewood Cliffs, NJ: Prentice Hall, 1987.

Wood W. Master Office Manual. Columbus, OH: Anadem Publishing, 1992.

ADDITIONAL READINGS

Becherer PD. A simple way to increase efficiency. Optometric Economics 2(5):31–34, 1992.

Borish IM. Delegation = survival. Optometric Economics 2(9):30–35, 1992.

Linkemer B. How to motivate your office staff. Optometric Economics 2(6):17–21, 1992.

Pride J. Employee performance problems: How to resolve them the right way. Journal of the American Dental Association 123:110–112, 1992.

Runninger J. You need a personnel manual. Optometric Economics 1(3):26–29, 1991.

Shelton L. Creating Teamwork. Boulder, CO: CareerTrack Publications, 1986.

Sullins WD Jr. Leadership in organized optometry. Journal of the American Optometric Association 62(7):509–510, 1991.

Part II

Applying Communication Techniques in the Clinic

12

Understanding the Patient's Experience

For a doctor to interact with patients effectively, it is important to be able to understand how patients experience disease and illness. It is also important to consider the factors that motivate patients to seek care as well as the factors that may prevent patients from adapting health-related behaviors. Without understanding the patient's experience, the doctor is at a significant disadvantage in interacting with patients and in working to identify appropriate intervention strategies.

DISEASE AND ILLNESS

It is estimated that at any given time, 75% to 90% of the population suffers from commonly encountered clinical symptoms, but that only one-third of these patients actually seek care (DiMatteo 1991). Why is it that some patients seek clinical care and others do not?

Patients often experience disease differently. Some report certain symptoms, while others describe different characteristics. This can occur because disease and illness are not exactly the same (Figure 12.1). Disease refers to the set of *clinical* signs such as examination results, clinical observations, and laboratory findings that indicate pathology. Illness refers to the set of *subjective* feelings that patients experience in response to pathology. Illness may involve physical, emotional, and psychological responses to disease.

Disease is the organ or system "breakdown." It is the element that is stressed in biomedical explanations. Illness is what the patient experiences

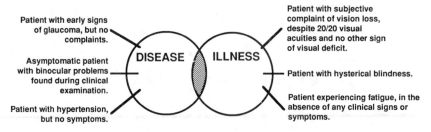

Patient with early signs of glaucoma, but no complaints.

Asymptomatic patient with binocular problems found during clinical examination.

Patient with hypertension, but no symptoms.

DISEASE   ILLNESS

Patient with subjective complaint of vision loss, despite 20/20 visual acuities and no other sign of visual deficit.

Patient with hysterical blindness.

Patient experiencing fatigue, in the absence of any clinical signs or symptoms.

Figure 12.1 Examples of disease and illness. Note the differences.

in response to clinical problems (Levenstein et al. 1989; Wright and Mac-Adam 1979; DiMatteo 1991).

It is possible to have disease without illness. This often occurs early in the course of a disease process, when clinical signs are evident but a patient is still asymptomatic (see Figure 12.1). This is frequently observed in patients who are newly diagnosed with early stage glaucoma. They experience no pain and discomfort, and they are usually not aware of visual field defects; however, if they are not treated for glaucoma, severe visual loss occurs.

Ms. Rodgens, a 59-year-old bank manager, presents for a general eye examination. Her uncorrected distance visual acuity is 20/20 in each eye. With a near correction of +2.00 O.U. she sees 20/20 in each eye. No visual symptoms are reported. The doctor finds that there is no change in her near prescription. No signs of binocular problems are found. Although other ocular health findings are unremarkable, the doctor finds cup-to-disc ratios of 0.65 in each eye, with intraocular pressures of 33 in the right eye and 29 in the left eye. The optic nerveheads and intraocular pressures are consistent with findings that suggest glaucoma. The patient reports absolutely no symptoms, yet, the doctor finds signs of pathology.

Mr. Caroll, a 31-year-old male, is a maintenance worker in a local park. He presents for a general eye examination with no symptoms. He is emmetropic, and all ocular health tests are negative. The doctor finds that he demonstrates a convergence insufficiency. Although clinical signs are evident to the doctor, the patient experiences no symptoms.

Mr. Ortero, a 64-year-old male, presents for a general eye examination. He works as an accountant. No ocular symptoms are present, and he has no history of ocular pathology. The optometrist finds uncorrected visual acuities of 20/20 in each eye at distance and 20/20 in each eye at near with a reading correction of +2.50 O.U. No binocular problems are found. Several flame-shaped hemorrhages, consistent with early background hypertensive retinopathy, are found in each eye. The patient's blood pressure is 165/95. The optometrist refers the patient to his internist who discusses the diagnosis of hypertension with Mr. Ortero. Although the patient is asymptomatic, clinical signs of disease are present.

In each of the three cases above, signs of pathology are present, but the patient experiences no symptoms. The contrasting situation (see Figure 12.1) can also occur. A patient may experience illness—the psychological experience of disease—in the absence of any noticeable clinical signs. Consider the following cases.

Ms. Hisario, a 37-year-old female, works as a journalist. She reports subjective complaints of vision loss over the past three months, but the doctor has not found any decrease in visual function. Visual acuity is 20/20 in each eye at distance and near. No signs of ocular pathology are present. Visual fields, contrast sensitivity, color vision, biomicroscopy, and ophthalmoscopic findings are all normal. Results of electrodiagnostic testing are also negative. No clinical findings indicating pathology are present; however, the patient perceives a decrease in the clarity of her vision.

Ms. Bower, a 13-year-old female, comes in for an eye examination. She complains of reduced vision in both eyes. You find that her best corrected visual acuity in her right eye is 20/400 and in her left eye is 20/200. A report from a previous eye doctor, from her old neighborhood, shows that her uncorrected visual acuity was 20/20 in each eye, at distance and near. Ocular health testing, including electrodiagnostic testing, is negative. A recent general examination at her pediatrician also uncovered no medical problems. The optometrist's discussion with the family reveals that the patient has been under a lot of stress in the past 8 months since the family moved to a new neighborhood. Her school work has also deteriorated since this move. No ocular basis for the decrease in vision is identified, and the optometrist identifies the problem as a case of hysterical blindness. Although there is no ocular basis for the problem, the symptoms are very real to the patient. The patient requires attention, and the optometrist recommends psychological counseling to help the patient handle some of the stress that she is experiencing.

Ms. Wachtman, a 49-year-old female, works as a librarian. Her best corrected visual acuity at distance, and near, is 20/20 in each eye. She has no visual symptoms. Ocular findings are also negative, with no sign of ocular pathology or binocular problems. She complains of fatigue and general weariness. A recent physical examination at her internist has revealed no medical problems or conditions, and she is not taking any medications. Extensive medical testing and investigation have revealed no indication of disease. The patient experiences fatigue, yet there are no clinical signs of disease.

These cases demonstrate that illness and disease do not always go together. Even when disease is accompanied by symptoms (Figure 12.1, shaded area) patients with the same diagnosis may have different symptoms, and their level of discomfort may vary. A one-to-one correspondence between disease and symptoms does not exist.

Why do different people experience disease and illness differently? One reason is that different people have different thresholds for pain and discomfort. Someone with a high threshold may not notice a problem until much later in the course of a disease. Individuals also respond differently to signs of illness. Some seek clinical care at the moment of onset of any physical symptoms of disease; others ignore signs unless they appear serious or advanced.

Patients tend to seek help (1) if they perceive their symptoms to be serious or important, (2) if they feel that their symptoms interfere enough with their ability to work or play, or (3) if others around them (e.g., relatives, friends, co-workers) are concerned about their symptoms and convince them to seek care. Triggers are the experiences that lead an individual to seek clinical care. Symptoms that serve as a trigger to one patient may not serve as a trigger to another.

If all patients with a particular diagnosis presented to the doctor's office with the same symptoms and complaints, diagnosis would be much easier. In reality, this is not the case. Some patients with retinal detachments present with certain symptoms, and some with others; still others present with no symptoms at all. It is up to the doctor to understand the patient's symptoms and perceptions, and to integrate them with clinical findings to evaluate the patient's experience.

THE BIOMEDICAL VERSUS BIOPSYCHOSOCIAL MODEL

A significant change in health care in recent years is the development of the biopsychosocial model of illness. The traditional biomedical model describes illness through explanations that are based *entirely* on biological changes that occur in the patient's body. The biopsychosocial model espouses that illness cannot be explained without considering the interactions that occur between biological, psychological, and social factors. Current attitudes in clinical care show a growing support for the biopsychosocial model as it is perceived to be more suitable in explaining health and illness.

THE LIFE CYCLE

The biopsychosocial model recognizes a combination of factors that influence a patient's health and well-being. At various ages individuals have different priorities and needs that can affect a patient's need for health care and responses to clinical intervention. The life cycle can be divided into a group of stages: infancy (birth to age 3), childhood (ages 3 to 11), adolescence (ages 11 to 18), young adulthood (ages 18 to 40), middle adulthood (ages 40 to 60), and later adulthood (age 60 and over).

Children and older patients utilize more health care services than adolescents and young adults (DiMatteo 1991). Children may need extra reassurance of their safety and security when brought into the clinical environment (see Chapter 16). Older individuals often have multiple health problems, and frequently have concerns about their continued health and well-being (see Chapter 13). Recognition of the patient's stage within the life cycle can enable the doctor to be more responsive to the patient's needs and priorities.

PATIENT'S RESPONSES TO DISEASE AND ILLNESS

Factors that affect a patient's *compliance* to medical recommendations have been described (see Chapter 7). These include family, friends, school or work environment, society, religion, culture, and previous experiences with the health care system. These factors are similar to those that affect a patient's *response* to medical problems. Whether patients decide to seek care for a particular problem and whether they fully express the magnitude of their symptoms and concerns to the doctor are often a factor of these influences.

Cultural responses to disease and clinical intervention will be discussed later in this chapter. Some patients are more likely to express pain and discomfort than others. Recent investigations have even shown gendered differences in communications (Tanenbaum 1990; Tannen 1990). Gender may affect how a patient expresses and responds to clinically significant signs.

The manner in which patients react to illness affects the way relatives, friends, co-workers, and health professionals respond to them and their probl

em. Some people are very hesitant to admit that they are sick, and resistant to physical limitations that result from illness. Others, however, react very positively to the advantages that accompany the "sick role." A patient who seeks minimal assistance may be treated differently from a family member who looks for bountiful care and attention. Health care professionals should be aware that family members' responses to illness may be affected by a patient's demonstration of the "sick role."

Sickness is sometimes used as a mechanism of controlling family activities and priorities. Illness can be used as a socially acceptable excuse for failing to meet one's responsibilities. The privileges and advantages of illness, often referred to as "secondary gains," can sometimes make it attractive (DiMatteo 1991).

CULTURAL RESPONSES TO SICKNESS
AND HEALTH CARE

Recent investigations have studied cultural influences on the utilization and responses to health care. Mumford (1985) identified differences in presenting complaints to health care practitioners. She mentions that in contrast to the English language, which has many words to describe pain (e.g., sharp, dull, throbbing), the language of the Navajo Indians has few words to indicate or describe pain; Navajos are culturally expected to "bear pain in silence." If Navajo patients do not express pain to a doctor it does not mean that they are not experiencing pain; it may just mean that they do not have the words to express their discomfort or that they do not believe that they are supposed to complain about their pain. As Mumford points out, some groups are more stoic in response to pain, and some are more open in expressing their symptoms.

To interact effectively with patients, the doctor has to be aware of cultural beliefs regarding health care. Folk beliefs about healing remedies and medicines frequently do not agree with standard medical and scientific practices. To ignore the fact that patients hold and follow these beliefs would make the doctor less effective in interacting with these patients and in designing useful management plans.

Some patients of Puerto Rican and Mexican-American background follow a "hot/cold theory of disease." This theory espouses that the body contains hot and cold "humors," and an adequate balance is required to maintain adequate health (Harwood 1971). Illness is believed to result from an imbalance between hot and cold "humors." Different diseases are identified as hot ("caliente") and cold ("frio"), and different medications and remedies are characterized as hot and cold. Arthritis and respiratory infections, for example, are classified as cold conditions; ulcers and skin eruptions are characterized as hot.

According to the theory, to restore the balance a "cold" illness is treated with a "hot" intervention. The doctor who inadvertently prescribes a hot remedy (e.g., a pill) for a hot disease would be inconsistent with the patient's belief systems, and would likely be met with resistance and noncompliance. Compliance in this situation is still attainable for the knowledgeable doctor who uses the principle of "neutralization." The patient can be told to take the hot remedy with a cold medium; thus, the patient concerned with the "hot/cold theory" can be told to take the pill with a cool drink. Doctors should be conscious of respecting cultural beliefs, and should not consider them to be unimportant. Only by being aware of and understanding the patient's belief systems can the doctor identify an effective intervention plan.

Another belief for many patients of Puerto Rican background is that an individual has only a fixed amount of blood that must last a lifetime; therefore, drawing blood for diagnostic purposes "diminishes" that individual

(Mumford 1985). The implications of recommending blood tests for individuals with these beliefs should be recognized.

It is believed that many Mexican-American patients prefer folk healers over traditional health care providers because their cultural healers are seen as more caring providers. When patients use prescribed medications, many of them discontinue treatment as soon as symptoms have decreased (DeSylvia-Valenti et al. 1992).

Some patients of Chinese background also consider health to be a balance of hot and cold energy forces ("yin" and "yang"). When an imbalance occurs, disease results; herbs are used to restore the balance (DeSylvia-Valenti et al. 1992).

Patients from different cultural backgrounds may also respond differently to use of touch in the clinical environment. In some cultures, touching is widely acceptable, and therapeutic touch would help put the patient at ease; in others, the doctor can make a patient uncomfortable by unnecessary contact.

Various cultures also have different styles of communication. As mentioned previously, the Navajo Indian has very few words to describe pain, and therefore may express minimal or no complaints about pain, even if it exists. Recent investigations have shown that men and women also have different styles of communication (Tanenbaum 1990; Tannen 1990) and different beliefs about their roles with respect to health care. Women use health care services more frequently than men, and they are more willing to express pain and discomfort (DiMatteo 1990). In 83% of homes across America, women are responsible for making medical and health-care decisions for themselves and their families (Tanenbaum 1990). Patients with different attitudes and beliefs regarding clinical care may respond to the health care system differently. Doctors who are most familiar with these characteristics are best prepared to meet the needs of their patients.

It is important to realize that not *all* patients of a particular cultural background subscribe to the "folk" practices associated with that culture. It is inappropriate—and potentially dangerous—to assume that individuals subscribe or adhere to cultural beliefs. The temptation to stereotype and categorize patients by ethnic and cultural beliefs should be avoided.

Doctors should also be aware that individuals may be familiar with "folk" practices of various cultures. Although many people are hesitant to share their cultural remedies with "outsiders," in some cases neighbors, friends, and co-workers share remedies. Patients have sometimes been introduced to health beliefs that would not seem likely, given their apparent ethnic and cultural background.

By being aware of folk remedies and healing practices of other cultures, health care professionals can recognize signs that indicate their presence and take positive steps to work effectively with patients to link gaps that occur between conventional clinical care and cultural practices. Inability to orient to the beliefs and customs of the patient can create a serious obstacle for the doctor in building compliance and mutual interaction.

Sometimes health care professionals can gain greater insights into cultural beliefs and "folk physiology" by calling in consultants who are familiar with these systems. Family members and other individuals from the same ethnic community as the patient ("cultural brokers") can help to clarify cultural health beliefs and identify treatment options that are mutually acceptable to the patient and doctor (DeSylvia-Valenti et al. 1992). The knowledgeable doctor can facilitate compliance by respecting the patient's beliefs and by working to identify appropriate intervention strategies.

PARALLEL AGENDA OF THE PATIENT AND DOCTOR

Levenstein and colleagues (1989) have suggested that when patients present for a clinical examination, there are two parallel agendas that have the potential to create misunderstanding (Figure 12.2). The goals of the doctor and patient may not be the same. The doctor is concerned with collecting a case history and gathering clinical findings that lead to a differential diagnosis. Patients are concerned with finding a cause for their problem and identifying a solution to allay their symptoms. Sometimes these parallel frameworks can proceed separately and create misunderstanding. The doctor, in an effort to gather clinical results, hurries from test to test. The patient, wondering why the doctor keeps bringing in new and complex instruments, assumes that the doctor must have found something bad. The patient becomes reserved and silent. The doctor wonders why the patient is not responding well to the tests.

Hopefully, this type of scenario is rare; however, it emphasizes the importance of orienting care to the patient. The doctor-oriented interview can help meet the goals of the doctor's agenda, but it may not meet the patient's goals and objectives in seeking clinical care. The most effective doctor can reconcile the differences across the two parallel agendas by delivering patient-centered care.

Remembering to respond to the patient as an *individual* is the basis of patient-oriented care. This approach is especially important in challenging situations such as working with the "difficult" patients discussed in Chapter 14. Appropriate use of language, effective development of doctor–patient rapport, insightful observation of nonverbal communications, and sensitive identification of the patient's needs and concerns can make the doctor more skillful in interacting with these patients. The doctor who is able to respond to each patient as an individual can be most successful in responding to the patient's individual needs, and in reconciling the parallel agendas of the doctor and patient.

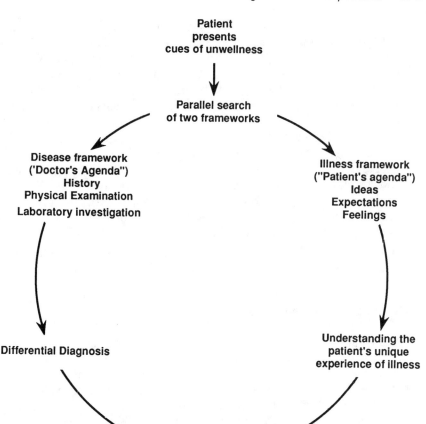

Figure 12.2 Parallel agendas of the doctor and patient. When patients present to the doctor, two parallel agendas exist. (Reprinted from Levenstein JH, Brown JB, Weston WW et al. Patient-centered interviewing. In Stewart M, Roter D, eds., Communicating with Medical Patients. Newbury Park, CA: Sage Publications, 1989, with permission.)

STRATEGIES FOR INTERACTING WITH PATIENTS EFFECTIVELY

To be effective, doctors must be able to understand the existence of clinical signs *and* the patient's experience of illness.

1. Remember that disease and illness are not always the same. A patient can experience disease without illness, and illness without disease. The

doctor who understands this distinction has achieved the first step in understanding a patient's perspective of clinical problems.

2. The traditional biomedical model describes illness as a result of biological changes in the patient's body. The biopsychosocial model encompasses a much broader range of factors that affect a patient's health status. Consider the wide range of factors that affect your patients' medical status.

3. To interact effectively with patients, doctors must recognize cultural beliefs and customs that affect health care. By understanding folk healing practices and systems, doctors can identify potential obstacles to compliance and address a patient's response to the health care delivery system.

4. When patients present to the clinical setting, doctors are often preoccupied with collecting information and making a differential diagnosis. Patients are generally interested in finding solutions to their problems. Effective doctors must be able to reconcile the differences that exist in these two agendas.

QUESTIONS FOR THOUGHT

1. You examine a patient who has cataracts in both eyes, resulting in best corrected visual acuities of 20/30 in each eye. This patient presented for a routine examination and has no complaints concerning ability to function. Another patient of the same age has the same type of lens changes, resulting in the same visual acuities. This patient has expressed strong complaints about both vision and the ability to function visually. Why would two patients report different levels of discomfort when they have identical clinical signs? How would you work with each patient to optimize compliance of your recommendations?

2. Give an example of a case in which a patient experiences disease without illness. Now give an example of a patient demonstrating illness without disease. Is it easier to build compliance in one category than in the other?

3. Make a list of factors that motivate patients to seek care when they experience a "red" eye. Now make a list of factors that motivate patients to seek care when they experience decreased vision. Are the factors the same, or are there differences?

4. Discuss the difference(s) between the biomedical and biopsychosocial models for a patient who has age-related macular degeneration (ARMD). Which do you think is more effective in explaining the experience of ARMD in patients?

5. Why would someone with a condition that results in impaired vision adapt a "sick role"? What types of questions can you ask to determine if a patient is trying to benefit from the advantages of a "sick role" status? If you observe signs, what can you do to assist the patient?

6. A patient presents to the doctor with a chief complaint of slightly blurred vision with the current reading prescription. The patient has no personal or family history of ocular disease. The doctor finds a mild change in the prescription that corresponds to the patient's visual symptoms, and, in addition, finds during the examination that the patient's tonometry readings are 32 (right eye) and 29 (left eye). Describe the agendas of the doctor and patient during this examination. What are the differences? How can these differences be reconciled?

REFERENCES

DeSylvia-Valenti DA, Good G, Mancil GL. Managing low income and minority elderly patients (Module 19). In Optometric Gerontology: A Resource Manual. Association of Schools and Colleges of Optometry, 6110 Executive Boulevard, Suite 514, Rockville, MD 20852, 1989. (Module 19, supplement added, 1992.)

DiMatteo MR. The Psychology of Health, Illness, and Medical Care. Pacific Grove, CA: Brooks/Cole, 1991.

Harwood A. The hot-cold theory of disease: Implications for the treatment of Puerto Rican patients. Journal of the American Medical Association 216:1153, 1971.

Levenstein JH et al. Patient-centered interviewing. In Stewart M, Roter D, eds., Communicating with Medical Patients. Newbury Park, CA: Sage Publications, 1989.

Mumford E. Culture: Life perspectives and the social meanings of illness. In Simons RC, ed., Understanding Human Behavior in Health and Illness. Baltimore, MD: Williams & Wilkins, 1985.

Tanenbaum J. Male and Female Realities: Understanding the Opposite Sex. San Marcos, CA: Robert Erdmann, 1990.

Tannen D. You Just Don't Understand: Women and Men in Conversation. New York: Ballantine Books, 1990.

Wright HJ, MacAdam DB. Clinical Thinking and Practice: Diagnosis and Decision in Patient Care. Edinburgh: Churchill Livingstone, 1979.

ADDITIONAL READINGS

Becker MH. Patient adherence to prescribed therapies. Medical Care 23:539–555, 1985.

Bernstein L, Bernstein RS. Interviewing: A Guide for Health Professionals. Norwalk, CT: Appleton-Century-Crofts, 1985.

Holman AM. Family Assessment: Tools for Understanding and Intervention. Newbury Park, CA: Sage Publications, 1983.

Payer L. Medicine and Culture. London: Penguin Books, 1988.

Smith RC, Hoppe RB. The patient's story: Integrating the patient- and physician-centered approaches to interviewing. Annals of Internal Medicine 115:470–477, 1991.

13

Optimizing Communication with Specific Patient Groups

This chapter will focus on optimal management of individuals from special patient groups including non-English-speaking, visually impaired, hearing impaired, geriatric, AIDS/HIV-positive, victims of childhood and adult domestic abuse, alcohol, drug, and substance abusers. These patients in particular can benefit from better doctor–patient communications and interactions. Each group has specific communication challenges; strategies for optimal management and intervention will be provided to help meet these challenges.

NON-ENGLISH-SPEAKING PATIENTS

Conducting examinations on patients who speak a foreign language is often challenging, particularly to clinical interns who are learning to perform the case history and clinical examination. Although communication in this type of situation may be difficult, the lack of a common language does not mean that communication is impossible. The clinician needs to be flexible and creative to discover ways of communicating effectively.

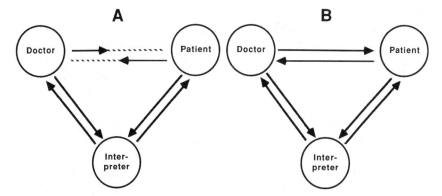

Figure 13.1 Communicating through an interpreter. When doctors examine patients who speak a foreign language, they must establish rapport with both the patient and the interpreter. Eye contact with both individuals must also be maintained.

Strategies for Interaction

1. Patients who speak a foreign language often bring interpreters with them to clinical examinations. If an interpreter is present, communication can be carried out by sending messages through the interpreter to the patient. The health care professional must be careful to develop rapport and maintain eye contact with the patient as well as the interpreter (see Chapters 1 and 6). There is often the temptation to look only at the interpreter and wait for the interpreter's translation of the patient's response. This may make the patient feel like a "nonperson" or child and should be avoided. Maintaining a proper balance of communication and appropriate eye contact with both the interpreter and the patient builds a more facilitative relationship (Figure 13.1).
2. Patients who speak a foreign language often have someone else call to make the appointment for them. It is helpful to ask the person calling if an interpreter can accompany the patient. By making the recommendation in advance, the patient can make arrangements to bring someone who can provide assistance.
3. Nonverbal cues are understood without the constraints of language. The doctor can communicate with gestures, facial expression, paralanguage, touch, and body language (Chapter 4). Use the patient's nonverbal cues to optimize communication.
4. It is an advantage to have bilingual staff members, especially if the practice is located in an area in which many residents speak a foreign language.

5. If the patient and the doctor do not share a common language, and an interpreter is not available, try to find areas of common understanding. Many patients who do not speak English are still able to read the letters on a Snellen chart, so visual acuity testing can still be performed. (Visual acuity charts for foreign languages are also available.) In addition, most patients can shake their head "yes" or "no" to indicate whether letters are clear or blurry.
6. Be creative in adapting other techniques for the examination when verbal communication is severely limited. If patients are not able to read letters, try using picture charts. Techniques such as the Broken Wheel test and Allen cards may be useful. In the end, the doctor may have to rely on objective tests, such as keratometry and retinoscopy, to obtain the desired information.
7. A common temptation in dealing with patients who speak a foreign language is to speak louder with the hope of getting the message across better. Health care professionals should remember that this does not help and may cause negative feelings in the patient. Flexibility, creativity, and patience can go a long way in handling these situations.
8. Patients who speak a foreign language are sometimes stereotyped as unintelligent because they cannot speak English. Doctors and their staff should be careful to treat these patients respectfully and kindly. What is a challenging situation for the professional should not have to result in an unpleasant encounter for the patient. All patients are entitled to warm, sensitive, competent care.

VISUALLY IMPAIRED PATIENTS

Several terms are used to describe changes in a patient's visual function. The doctor who understands these terms and their distinctions can be helpful to the patient who is trying to cope with vision loss (Freeman 1991; Lovie-Kitchin and Bowman 1985).

> A *visual impairment* is a *limitation of function* that is not correctable by standard methods; decreases in visual acuity, contrast sensitivity, and dark adaptation resulting from macular degeneration are examples.
> A *visual disability* is a *limitation in the ability to perform certain tasks*. A disability can result from a decreased function. For example, a decrease in visual acuity can affect a patient's abilities in reading, writing, watching television, and recognizing faces.
> A *visual handicap* is a *patient's perceived disadvantage* that occurs as a result of a disability. If patients believe that they can no longer read or write because of a disability, then they perceive that they are handicapped in these areas.

Freeman (1991) recommends shifting the focus of the discussion with patients and their families from visual handicaps to looking at visual disabilities. By considering disabilities, and not concentrating extensively on handicaps, patients can attend to setting goals and working with low vision aids that can improve function.

> Mr. Barton is a 64-year-old male who has worked as a copyeditor for a publisher for the past 39 years. Proliferative diabetic retinopathy has decreased the vision in his right eye at distance to 20/40 and his left eye to 20/60. Mr. Barton indicates to the doctor that he enjoys his job, and takes great pride in the quality of his work over the last 39 years. He says that he feels that he has to "give it up" soon because his vision has prevented him from performing his editing responsibilities adequately. His perceived disadvantage from his visual problems has caused him a great deal of anguish. By identifying Mr. Barton's visual disability at work, the doctor can begin to discuss low vision aids and devices that can be of assistance in the editing activities.

Knowing how to deliver clinical services in a caring manner is an essential characteristic for the low vision practitioner. When first confronted with vision loss, patients often need assistance in learning to adapt to changes in their visual function. Family members may also need supportive communications.

It is important for patients, family members, and doctors to arrive at realistic goals and expectations for low vision care. Many patients and their families want the doctor to restore their vision to the way it was before the loss. Unrealistic expectations can hinder hopes for success. By discussing alternatives with patients and their families, the doctor can choose optimal rehabilitation strategies that meet the patient's needs.

> Ms. Heyward is a 61-year-old female who works as a department store administrator. She presents to the optometrist's office with complaints of reduced vision at distance and near over the past three to five months. She is particularly concerned about her reading abilities. She has a history of hypertension over the past 5 years and takes Procardia and is monitored by her internist regularly. She has a history of myopia and astigmatism, but no history of visual problems or pathology. There is no family history of ocular disease.
>
> Dr. Jentsen examines her and finds that she has age-related macular degeneration. Pigmentary changes and atrophy of the retinal pigment epithelium are present in the maculae of both eyes; no fluid or hemorrhages are present, but scattered drusen are observed in the macular region of both eyes. The patient's best corrected acuity is 20/70 in the right eye and 20/50 in the left eye, at distance and near. The patient was able to read 20/20 in each eye several years ago, and is unhappy with the current clarity of her vision.

> DR. JENTSEN: Ms. Heyward, as I have explained to you, I have found that you have what is called age-related macular degeneration. That means that there have been some changes in the area of your retina that is responsible for the clearest vision. When this area of the retina is disturbed, it results in decreased vision.

That's why you have noticed that your vision has not been as clear as it used to be.

MS. HEYWARD: Are you going to give me new glasses?

DR. JENTSEN: Yes, I am going to give you a new prescription for glasses, but I want to make sure that you understand that these glasses will not restore your vision to what it used to be. It will make you see as well as you are able to *now*, but it will not give you the same level of vision that you used to have.

MS. HEYWARD: Well, can't you give me a different pair of glasses or some drops to take? (The patient is trying to find a cure for her problem, and is not happy with the limitation that remains.)

DR. JENTSEN: Unfortunately, the problem that we are talking about is not one that can be corrected by glasses or drops. I understand your desire to see clearly and your concern about having good vision. (The doctor responds to the patient's affective level and her concerns.) The type of degeneration on your retina is not one that is reversible, so I don't expect your clearest vision to return. (The doctor proceeds to provide the patient with more factual information about her condition.) What we can do is watch your eyes very carefully from now on. It's very important to pick up certain types of changes that can occur, to prevent further vision loss. I would be happy to answer any questions that you have. (As the patient expresses a readiness to learn more, the doctor explains more about using an Amsler grid, and maintaining regular follow-up visits. By providing the patient with facts, sensitivity, and a realistic explanation, the doctor helps the patient understand her situation.)

Patients should realize that rehabilitation is often slow and that it requires work and practice on the part of the patient, the doctor, and caretakers.

Strategies for Interaction

1. Be sensitive to patients' attitudes and feelings in response to vision loss. Losing sensory function often leads to periods of bereavement or mourning for the lost function. Patients may feel shock, denial, anger, grief, depression, or acceptance. They may experience feelings of helplessness, lowered self-esteem, and diminished independence.
2. Be aware of factors that affect the patient's self-image. Shindell (1988) explains that low vision is not the type of problem that easily lends itself to rapid understanding and support from other people because it is an "invisible" problem. There are usually no external scars, and no visible signs or indications. Relatives may wonder why an individual cannot work, and co-workers may wonder why a person is unable to perform certain functions. Understanding can be difficult for patients, as well as their relatives and co-workers.

3. A recommended format for the low vision interview is provided in Appendix B.5. The actual interview can be more conversational and less structured, but the basic categories should all be addressed.
4. Goals can change during adaptation. Cole (1991) recommends that patients be asked about their goals at least three times during the first visit: at the beginning and end of the case history, and again at the end of the first visit. Goals should be discussed again at follow-up visits.
5. Encourage patients to take active roles in the rehabilitation process. It is believed that feelings of self-control and determination are important for rehabilitation (Shute 1991).
6. Be particularly sensitive when approaching the task of educating patients about low vision devices. The patient has to be ready in all three learning dimension areas: cognitive, psychomotor, and affective (see Chapter 8).
7. Educate the patient on the types of optical and nonoptical aids that are available. Provide the opportunity for the patient to see and try various lenses, magnifiers, telescopes, microscopes, and nonoptical aids. Trying different aids and devices will help patients determine what works best for them. During training, educate the patient about magnification, field of view, appropriate working distances, and lighting. Mehr and Fried (1975) suggest that a patient should know what a finished low vision aid looks like *before* it is ordered.
8. A patient's acceptance of a low vision device depends on a number of factors including comfort, flexibility of the device, cost, appearance of the system in public, availability of the device, and perceived success. Many patients are resistant to low vision aids, such as telescopic systems that are very noticeable in public. Some patients are more receptive to hand and stand magnifiers, which provide easy mobility and can be used and easily removed from view.
9. Educational materials should be printed with letters that are large enough for patients with decreased vision to read (Freeman and Jose 1991).
10. Low vision practitioners and staff should be attentive to the patient's emotional responses to vision loss. Counseling and appropriate referrals to psychologists, social workers, and psychiatrists are essential when a response such as extreme depression is observed.
11. Assess the patient's needs across several categories: primary and secondary needs, activities of daily living, and instrumental activities of daily living. Primary needs include communication (written and spoken), mobility, home and personal management, and emotional/psychological needs. Secondary needs include recreation, socialization, accommodation, financial, vocational education, health care, and community integration (Lovie-Kitchin and Bowman 1985).

Functions can also be divided into two categories: activities of daily living (ADL) such as eating, bathing, grooming, toileting, ambulation, and transportation; and instrumental activities of daily living (IADL), which allow patients to maintain independent community living. The latter category includes managing finances, shopping, using public transportation, and using the telephone.

12. Help patients to adapt to changes in their environment and lives. Life-change events such as the death of a spouse, divorce, moving, changing jobs, change in working conditions, and change in social activities can all affect an individual's level of stress, health, and life style (Holmes and Rahe 1967). These life-change events can result in even more significant changes in their ability to function and cope. A change in employment or job conditions may require patients to use their eyes differently. Death of a spouse may mean that there is no one available to help read the mail or to handle the family finances. The optometrist who has a long-term relationship with a patient can be instrumental in helping the patient adjust to major life-change events.

13. Members of the office staff may be asked to assist in training activities or answer questions about the use of low vision aids on the telephone or in the office. Staff members' attitudes toward patients with low vision, and the use of low vision aids, can have a significant impact on the patient's progress and adaptation.

14. Providing low vision services requires extra time. Schedule your appointments appropriately.

15. Make the patient aware of community resources and local services such as counseling, vocational rehabilitation, educational programs, health care services, and sources of low vision products (e.g., large print watches, playing cards, publications, and books on tape).

PATIENTS WITH HEARING IMPAIRMENTS

Hearing impairments can be congenital or acquired. They can result from injuries and diseases that affect the auditory system, prolonged exposure to loud noises, degenerative processes, and ototoxic effects from certain drugs (Weinstein 1989). Hearing loss is especially prominent in the elderly population; up to 60% of individuals over 65 experience some degree of hearing impairment (Weinstein 1989). Hearing impairments are often undetected and unidentified; undetected hearing problems can be misidentified as cognitive, affective, or psychiatric disorders (Weinstein 1989; Weinstein 1990).

Many patients with hearing deficits are fit with hearing aids. Assistive listening devices (ALDs), such as telephone amplifiers, involve a microphone, amplifier, and receiver to enhance sound. Electronic devices are readily available, and some health care professionals keep electronic amplifying systems available to use with hearing-impaired patients.

The need for good eye care for hearing-impaired individuals should be emphasized as part of maximizing a person's abilities. Hearing loss can have a significant impact on an individual's daily living activities. If a significant refractive error remains uncorrected, a secondary visual disability is imposed on an already disadvantaged patient (see Chapter 17). To maximize visual skills and abilities, good eye care is imperative.

Sensory deficits, such as hearing impairments, can create an obstacle to effective communication in the clinical environment. Strategies for working with hearing-impaired individuals depend greatly on the intensity and type of problem. Orienting to the individual needs of the patient leads to a more therapeutic interaction and effective care.

Strategies for Interaction

1. Learn to identify patients with hearing deficits. Patients who speak very loudly, who frequently ask you to repeat what you have said, and who seem to miss parts of oral communications may be demonstrating a hearing loss. Some patients conspicuously lip-read but are unaware that they do so. Since not all patients realize that they have a hearing difficulty, and some choose to ignore or deny the problem, the health care provider should be observant of signs and indicators.
2. The questions in Table 13.1 may be helpful in determining whether a patient has a hearing impairment. When a hearing deficit is suspected

Table 13.1 Screening inventory for hearing loss

1. Do you feel embarrassed or frustrated when you can't hear what people say?
2. Does your hearing cause you to feel frustrated when talking to members of your family?
3. Do you have difficulty hearing when someone speaks in a whisper?
4. Do you feel handicapped by a hearing problem?
5. Do you have a problem hearing when visiting friends, relatives, or neighbors?
6. Does a hearing problem cause you to attend religious services less often than you would like?
7. Does a hearing problem cause you to have arguments with family members?
8. Do you find that people comment on the volume of your TV or radio?
9. Do you feel that any difficulty with your hearing limits or hampers your personal or social life?
10. Do you have a problem hearing relatives or friends when in a restaurant or crowded area?
11. Do you find it easier to hear on one side or the other?

Modified from Ventry I, Weinstein B. Identification of elderly people with hearing problems. American Speech-Language-Hearing Association (ASHA) July:37–42, 1983.

and the patient has not been evaluated, referral for audiologic testing is indicated.

3. When examining a hearing impaired patient, try to establish how the patient communicates as early as possible in the clinical interview.

   For patients who lip-read, face the patient directly, and speak at a reasonably normal speed. It may be helpful to slow down your speech a little, but lipreaders are used to reading at a regular pace, so slowing down excessively may impede a reader's understanding. Be certain that there is adequate lighting so the patient can see your lips. When testing must be performed in the dark, it is helpful to give the patient directions before the lights are turned out, or to raise the illumination again during testing if additional instructions to the patient are required.

4. Stand on the patient's "better" side; patients will often tell you which is their "better" side. If both ears are affected equally, and the patient has only one hearing aid, stand on the side of the patient with the hearing aid.

5. Consider learning American Sign Language (ASL) or finger spelling to improve your capacity for communication. Staff members may also be interested in learning these techniques.

6. Consider installing a Telecommunication Device for the Deaf (TDD) in your office. This instrument allows hearing-impaired individuals to call your office to make appointments. With the TDD, the verbal communication is typed to the patient's machine from the one in your office, so the hearing-impaired individual can "see" the conversation.

7. Be aware that especially with hearing-impaired individuals, nonverbal communications can strengthen and enhance the delivery of information.

8. Monitor the patient's understanding—use "checking" questions (see Chapter 2) to verify. Provide corrective feedback when necessary.

9. If verbal communications are difficult, try written instructions. For example, the patient may prefer writing the letters that they see on a Snellen chart, rather than saying them aloud.

10. Be attentive to the patient's preferred form of communication, and try to incorporate the patient's preferences into your methods of testing.

11. Schedule adequate time for working with these patients as they often require more time than normally allotted for a regular examination.

12. Patient education activities should include pictures, models of the eye, and written directions. With hearing-impaired individuals, use of vision and touch can be particularly helpful (see Chapter 8).

GERIATRIC PATIENTS

One of eight Americans is 65 years of age or older. It is estimated that by the year 2020, 15% to 20% of Americans will be 65 or older (Optometric Gerontology 1989; Shute 1991).

The aging population presents some new challenges to the health care delivery system. Research and investigations in gerontology (the study of aging) and geriatrics (the discipline of caring for the elderly who are sick) have increased in recent years.

Many health care providers are under the impression that most older individuals are sick, weak, and away in nursing homes. A large proportion of older individuals are able to take care of their own needs, and many lead very active lives. Only 5% suffer from severe senile dementia and only 5% live in nursing homes. Stereotyping and negative attitudes about aging (agism) are obstacles to effective care for older individuals. A better understanding of aging can help to eliminate stereotypes and biases and prepare health care professionals to help older patients.

Aging is accompanied by various physical, physiological, sensory, and motor changes. Understanding these changes can enable the eye care professional to become better prepared to provide care to older patients. Changes in the patient's reaction time, memory, and psychomotor skills may all affect the doctor's choices and modes of testing and intervention. "Normal" aging changes include increased neural conduction rates resulting in slowed reaction time, decreased muscle strength, decreased bone mass, decreased speed of learning, and some decrease in memory (visual memory appears to decline more rapidly than auditory memory [Weinman 1987]).

Eighty-five percent of older individuals suffer from at least one chronic physical condition (DiMatteo 1991). Conditions such as arthritis, rheumatism, heart disease, and strokes occur at higher rates than in younger populations. Older individuals also have a high prevalence of multiple health problems.

Presbycusis, hearing loss associated with aging, tends to occur gradually and is usually bilateral and symmetrical. Age-related hearing loss occurs in both the low and high frequencies, with a greater loss in the high-frequency range. Up to 60% of individuals over 65 experience some degree of hearing impairment. Most of these are mild to moderate losses, with only about 10% to 15% identified as severe or profound (Weinstein 1989).

Almost one of six Americans of age 65 or older is blind or severely visually impaired. Several of the major causes of blindness are age-related: macular degeneration, cataracts, glaucoma, diabetic retinopathy, and hypertensive retinopathy. The increasing aging population indicates that more professionals are needed to care for the visual demands of older individuals.

Mr. Harper is an 82-year-old male who presents to Dr. Fuentes' office for the first time. His 58-year-old daughter accompanies him to the examination and describes him as a "complainer." "He doesn't like doctors," she warns Dr. Fuentes. The patient's last eye examination was 4 years ago. He was diagnosed with "early cataracts" but has no history of any other ocular problems or disease. He has hypertension and has been treated with antihypertensives since age 61. No other medical problems are known.

Dr. Fuentes starts out by shaking the patient's hand, and greeting him warmly. (The doctor is trying to establish a safe and secure environment for the patient.) He tells the patient that he is going to examine his eyes and check his vision today. "If you have any questions as we go along," he says to the patient, "feel free to let me know and I will try to answer any questions you have." He notices that the patient takes some time to respond during the case history, so he allows extra time for the patient to respond during the rest of the case history and examination sequence. By not rushing the patient, and providing the time needed, the doctor creates a relaxed atmosphere that is conducive to participation. The doctor notices that the patient speaks loudly. He observes that when he speaks at a normal tone, the patient tends to ask him to repeat the question. To communicate more effectively, the doctor tries to speak loudly to meet the patient's need. The doctor inquires whether there is any history of hearing problems. The patient and the daughter say that they are not aware of any, but the daughter says that he has been speaking "louder and louder" and often misses parts of what is said.

From his examination, the doctor finds that the patient has advancing cataracts (moderate nuclear sclerosis and anterior cortical changes, both eyes). The patient's function is not disturbed significantly, and surgical intervention is not deemed necessary at this time. New glasses for distance and reading are prescribed to help the patient function better. Dr. Fuentes reminds the patient to continue following the status of the hypertension with his internist. He also recommends audiological testing since the patient manifests signs of hearing loss and has never been tested.

Throughout the examination, the doctor is conscious of building a rapport with both the patient and his daughter. This helps lead to a productive and successful interaction.

Strategies for Interaction

1. Older patients may take longer to process information. When indicated, it is often helpful to speak a little slower and to allow more time for patients to respond.
2. Speak louder around patients who are hearing impaired. Written instructions can also enhance understanding. (See the previous section on hearing-impaired patients for additional strategies.)
3. When a new drug therapy is given, consider possible drug interactions with other prescribed drugs and over-the-counter medications that the patient is taking. The doctor should also make sure that patients do not discontinue other unrelated drug therapies.
4. Provide forms and patient handouts in large print.

5. Causes of noncompliance in the elderly may include loss of memory, poor understanding of instructions, confusion with multiple medical regimens, and inability to comply (e.g., can't afford medications, no one to bring them for follow-up appointments, can't open childproof caps). To minimize nonadherence:

   a. Provide written take-home instructions to reinforce a patient's memory of directions and instructions.

   b. If labels on containers and bottles of medications are small, provide the patient with a copy of the directions in advance, in larger print. (A patient who cannot read the label may not take the medication at the appropriate times.)

   c. If patients have motor problems or decreased muscle strength, suggest that they ask the pharmacist to avoid using childproof caps with their prescriptions.

6. Provide supportive communications and respond to affective as well as cognitive messages. Older individuals frequently experience major losses and adverse life changes such as the death of relatives and friends, changes in health, financial changes, and modifications in employment and social activities. They may have to adjust to impaired functions such as decreased vision and hearing.

7. Be alert to signs of depression in the elderly. These signs include apathy, fatigue, anxiety, sleep disturbances, loss of interest, loss of weight, and decreased self-esteem. Referrals to psychological and psychiatric colleagues can help these patients deal more effectively with life changes.

8. Avoid negative stereotypes of older people. Consider each patient's individual abilities and needs.

PATIENTS WITH AIDS AND HIV INFECTION

The emergence of acquired immune deficiency syndrome (AIDS) has had a significant impact on the health of people across the country and on the delivery of health care. The serious nature of the disease and the difficulty in treating patients with human immunodeficiency virus (HIV) infection evoke strong emotional responses. Many sensitive issues can arise, and many of these require refined interpersonal effectiveness and sensitivity.

As a result of the emergence of AIDS, health professionals in a variety of clinical specialty areas now find it necessary to become confident and comfortable in taking sexual histories, and in addressing issues that relate to sexuality.

Most of the components of the sexual history relate to the occurrence of risky behaviors that are associated with the transmission of HIV disease and other sexually transmitted diseases. Table 13.2 shows the types of questions that the health care professional may want to consider asking. In

Table 13.2 Case history questions on sexuality

Are you sexually active?

Do you practice "safe sex"?

Have you had multiple sexual partners?

Do you engage in unprotected sex with any individuals who are in high-risk groups (e.g., IV drug users, individuals with multiple sexual partners)?

Have you ever been diagnosed with a sexually transmitted disease (such as syphilis, herpes, or gonorrhea)?

Have you ever been diagnosed as being HIV-positive?

Have any of your partners been diagnosed as being HIV-positive?

Do you engage in any high-risk behaviors (e.g., sharing needles with IV drug abusers, engaging in sexual relations with unknown or multiple partners)?

Do you have any concerns about having any sexually transmitted diseases, such as AIDS?

Is there anything else on this topic that you would like to discuss?

addition to the sexual history, health care professionals concerned about AIDS should also inquire about whether the patient has ever shared needles with other individuals (e.g., in drug abuse). For issues on sexuality that fall beyond the expertise of the eye care professional, referrals to general physicians, gynecologists, urologists, and therapists who specialize in sexual disorders and human sexuality may be indicated.

Patients do not always identify themselves as HIV-positive to doctors. Many are concerned about discriminatory effects if others find out about their status, and some are worried that doctors will be afraid to take care of them. Doctors should be aware of the signs and symptoms of HIV-positive individuals and should encourage honest, open disclosures to ensure optimal care. Sometimes ensuring the patient of the confidentiality of a patient's record and information is helpful.

Mr. Byrne is a 39-year-old male who presents to the optometrist's office for a routine examination. He expresses no visual complaints, and except for a report of conjunctivitis two years ago, his ocular history is unremarkable. He says that he is in good general health, not taking any medications, or being followed for any medical problems. He mentions only that he occasionally gets seasonal allergies, and that "over-the-counter" pills eliminate his symptoms.

As the optometrist prepares to do ophthalmoscopy and explains that the back of his eye will be looked at, the following conversation occurs:

Dr. Harred: Mr. Byrne, I'm going to shine a light in the back of your eyes now to make sure that they are nice and healthy.

MR. BYRNE: Can you tell if a patient has cytomegalovirus (CMV) when you look with that light?

(The doctor is surprised by this sudden question and considers the possibility that the patient is HIV-positive. CMV retinitis is one of the ocular manifestations of HIV disease. Most patients do not know about CMV unless they have had some experience with it or have heard about it. Dr. Harred decides that it is worth proceeding to find out if CMV retinitis is a personal concern for the patient.)

DR. HARRED: When we look in the back of the eye, we are able to see signs of CMV retinitis. Is this something that is of concern to you?

MR. BYRNE: No, I was just wondering about it.

DR. HARRED: OK, that's fine. I just want to make sure that it is not a personal concern for you. Many people with HIV disease are concerned about CMV retinitis. When patients are HIV-positive, it is important for the doctor to know, so optimal care can be provided. Have you ever tested positive for HIV, or is HIV a concern for you?

MR. BYRNE: Well, . . . (The patient hesitates but doesn't continue.)

(The doctor can tell that there is something on the patient's mind, and wants to encourage him to speak openly with her.)

DR. HARRED: Mr. Byrne, I want to assure you that our records are completely confidential. No one has access to them, and I do not discuss my patients' information with anyone else, unless they ask me to. To give you the best care, it is important for me to have all of the information about your health. Is there anything further that you would like to discuss?

MR. BYRNE: Well, . . . yes, I found out that I am HIV-positive a few years ago, and I am very concerned about that.

DR. HARRED: I can understand how you must feel. (The doctor responds to the patient's affective statement.) That must be a difficult situation. Do you remember when you first found out?

MR. BYRNE: Yes, it was about three years ago.

DR. HARRED: How has your health been since then?

MR. BYRNE: It's been fine. I've really been in excellent health. No problems. No signs at all.

DR. HARRED: Have you been treated with any medications?

MR. BYRNE: No, my doctor has not put me on any medications at this point.

DR. HARRED: Have you been following up with your doctor regularly?

MR. BYRNE: Yes, I go to the clinic every few months.

DR. HARRED: I'm glad that you decided to discuss this with me, Mr. Byrne. I want to assure you that what we have discussed is confidential, and that it will allow me to give you the best care. (The doctor provides reassurance to the patient for an open disclosure, and the examination continues in a supportive environment.)

Strategies for Interaction

1. Be sensitive in dealing with the emotional issues that affect patients with HIV disease. Do not avoid the affective cues that patients project, and respond only to the clinical/scientific issues.
2. Create a warm, supportive environment for patients, free of biases.
3. Be familiar with sensitive ways of discussing bad news and providing supportive communication (see Chapter 5).
4. Strive to gain competence and comfort in taking a sexual history and in inquiring about issues that relate to sexuality. When indicated, referrals to other health care professionals who deal more directly with sexual function can be made.
5. Stay up to date on the rapidly expanding scientific and clinical knowledge base on AIDS by reading relevant journal articles and books and attending clinical programs that address this topic.

CHILD AND ADULT DOMESTIC ABUSE

Over 1.5 million children across the country were reported as abused and neglected during a recent one-year period (Kessler and Hyden 1991). Ocular manifestations occur in approximately 40% of physically abused children (Smith 1988). Thirty-three percent of injuries to adult domestic violence victims occur to the face and neck (New York State Office for the Prevention of Domestic Violence 1990). Child abuse and adult domestic violence are widespread problems in this country. Eye care professionals can serve an important function in recognizing signs of physical abuse and taking appropriate steps.

The initial "communication" of problems is usually through clinical signs such as bruises, injuries, and lacerations; victims of violence rarely claim that they have been abused. The perceptive health care professional must follow up with inquiries about the origin of the injuries. Through effective interviewing, health care providers can obtain disclosures. Once a disclosure is made, the doctor can encourage the patient to take positive steps to address the problem. It is often challenging to get disclosures, because both children and adults usually are afraid of "squealing" on anyone. Facilitative questioning and empathic responding are helpful.

Because it is easier, health care professionals tend to treat symptoms, rather than underlying causes of physical abuse. However, treating only the symptoms (e.g., the black eyes) without investigating the underlying causes (e.g., battering) perpetuates the cycle of abuse. Until recently, most health care professionals were not trained to identify and handle cases of child and domestic abuse.

Child Abuse

Child abuse includes physical and sexual abuse, maltreatment, and neglect. Physical abuse occurs when a child suffers from nonaccidental injuries that are inflicted by a parent or an adult who is responsible for the child. Maltreatment and neglect occur when a child is subjected to impaired physical, mental, or emotional conditions. The parent may not supply the child with adequate food, clothing, shelter, education, medical care, or may expose the child to substantial risk or harm.

Although the laws may differ, all 50 states require mandated reporting of suspected child abuse by health care professionals, including optometrists and ophthalmologists. "Suspected" means that the doctor does not have to be certain that child abuse exists; if there is reason to suspect abuse, then the doctor is obligated to report the case. Investigations are then conducted to confirm or rule out the suspicions of abuse.

Strategies for Interaction

1. Be observant of signs of child abuse: bruises, lacerations, welts, bite marks, burns, fractures, and head injuries. These should serve as "red flags" for the clinician to suspect abuse. Table 13.3 lists primary and secondary ocular signs of child abuse. Primary factors are usually indicators of child abuse, unless other reasonable explanations are available. Intraocular hemorrhages in children aged two and under are especially suggestive of child abuse, unless proven otherwise (Smith 1988). Secondary factors are sometimes associated with abuse; further inquiry and observations can provide additional insights. Emotional and behavioral signs of child abuse are identified in Table 13.4.
2. Be aware of the patterns of physical abuse.
   a. Bilateral patterns of injury. Accidental injury is usually unilateral. When people fall they tend to fall on one side, so injuries are usually limited to that side: one arm, one leg, one side of the face. When people are beaten, they are often hit on both sides of the body or face.
   b. Multiple signs of injury. Unexplained injury to multiple areas can be a sign of abuse. Injuries to the face and arms, in the absence of satisfactory explanations, warrant further investigation.
   c. Repeated episodes of injury. If a parent brings a child in for multiple office visits, with repeated physical injuries, further investigation is indicated.
   d. Injuries that are inconsistent with a parent's explanation indicate a need for further inquiry. If a child has rope burns, and the parent says the child fell, or if the parent dates the injury inconsistently with the color of the bruises, suspicion should be raised.

Table 13.3 Ocular signs of child abuse

Primary signs[a]	Intraocular hemorrhages
	Preretinal hemorrhage
	Retinal hemorrhage
	Vitreous hemorrhage
	Subretinal hemorrhage
Secondary signs[b]	Retinal detachments/dialysis
	Hyphema
	Hypopeon
	Iritis/iridodialysis
	Periorbital edema/ecchymosis
	Angle recession
	Blowout fracture
	Ptosis
	Proptosis
	Strabismus
	Dislocated/subluxated lens
	Cataracts
	Retinal tears
	Glaucoma
	Disconjugate ocular motilities
	Corneal edema/scars
	Subconjunctival edema/scars
	Subconjunctival hemorrhages
	Choroidal rupture/scar/atrophy
	Anisocoria/pupillary anomalies
	Papilledema
	Purtscher's retinopathy
	Lid lacerations
	Penetrating/perforating wounds
	Chemical burns
	Eyelid crab louse infestation
	Cortical blindness
	Ruptured globe

[a]Primary signs should be considered signs of suspected child abuse in very young children, unless proven otherwise.
[b]Secondary signs may indicate the occurrence of child abuse; further investigation is needed to evaluate the situation.

Modified with permission from Smith SK. Child abuse and neglect: A diagnostic guide for the optometrist. Journal of the American Optometric Association 59(10):760–766, 1988.

    e. Varied explanations. It is best to interview the child separately from the parents; it may be helpful to interview each parent separately as well. Look for inconsistencies in the stories of all related parties.

Table 13.4 Emotional/behavioral indicators of child abuse

Apprehensive of contact with parents and other adults
Fearful of strangers
Low self-esteem
Running away from home
General failure to thrive
Poor school performance
Poor school attendance
Behavior problems
Sleeping problems
Self-injurious behaviors (e.g., suicidal thoughts and attempts)
Withdrawal from other children and adults
Aggressiveness
Drug/alcohol/substance abuse
Display of sexual promiscuity/acting out

Modified with permission from Smith SK. Child abuse and neglect: A diagnostic guide for the optometrist. Journal of the American Optometric Association 59(10):760–766, 1988.

One parent's story may seem to change as the parent is asked to repeat the story a few times.

   f. Multiple stages of bruising. Multiple bruises at different stages of healing suggest that they were incurred at different times. Colors of bruising suggest the time that has occurred since injury (Fleisher and Ludwig 1988; Kessler and Hyden 1991) (see Table 13.5).

3. Build trust in the child—eye contact and therapeutic touch can help. Assure children that you will not discuss their responses with the parent.

4. When disclosures are difficult to obtain, or information is conflicting, ask questions in different words.

5. Remember that children and parents involved in cases of child abuse are often confused and afraid. They need a supportive environment and a caring health provider.

Table 13.5 Color of bruising in relation to time occurred since injury

Color	*Time Since Injury*
Red, reddish blue	0–24 hours
Purple, dark blue	1–4 days
Greenish, yellow-green	5–7 days
Yellow, brown	7–14 days
Normal tint (bruise disappears)	1–3 weeks

6. Be familiar with appropriate procedures for reporting child abuse in your state.
7. Be aware of local resources and services that can help parents and children. Counseling services, local support groups, and agencies can provide information and assistance.

Adult Domestic Violence

Adult domestic violence involves patterns of physical, sexual, psychological, emotional, and/or economic abuse. These behaviors are exerted by one family member over another, with the goal of establishing and maintaining power and control. A five-pronged wheel (Figure 13.2) has been used to demonstrate the behaviors that constitute domestic abuse (New York State Office for the Prevention of Domestic Violence 1990). It is important to realize that a person does not have to be physically injured to be a victim of domestic abuse. Psychological, emotional, and economic abuse involve patterns of behavior that are harmful and injurious.

Ninety-five percent of adult domestic violence cases involve female victims injured by male partners, either married or unmarried; less than 5% of cases involve female abusers and male victims. An act of adult domestic violence occurs every 15 seconds, more frequently than any other crime in the country. Battering is the single major cause of injury to women in the country, more frequent than automobile accidents, muggings, and rapes combined (New York State Office for the Prevention of Domestic Violence 1990).

Ms. Marlowe is a 45-year-old female who presents to the optometrist's office complaining of a "black eye." There is periorbital ecchymosis and conjunctival injection seen on gross observation. The following interaction takes place during the case history.

Dr. Bradley: Ms. Marlowe, I see that you have a "black eye." How did it occur?

Ms. Marlowe: A box hit me in the eye.

Dr. Bradley: How did you get hit with a box? (The doctor tries to establish how the incident occurred.)

Ms. Marlowe: I was sitting on my chair, and a box hit me in my eye. (The patient appears very reticent to discuss the incident.)

Dr. Bradley: Ms. Marlowe, is there someone who threw the box? Boxes don't hit someone on their own. There is usually someone behind them. Who threw the box? (The doctor issues a confronting question, after trying to get the information in other more subtle ways.)

Ms. Marlowe: (Hesitantly) ... The box just hit me. (At this point, the doctor feels that the patient is not ready to open up and decides to proceed with the examination and to return to the issue of the box later.)

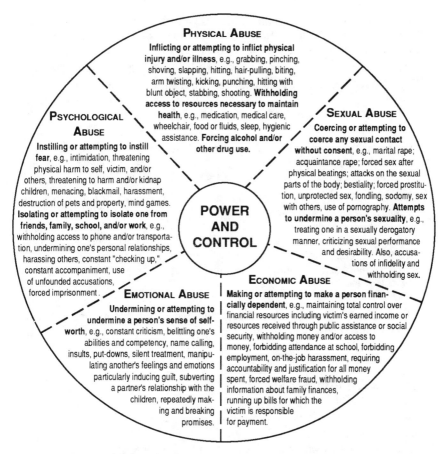

Figure 13.2 Power and control perspective of domestic violence. Domestic violence involves patterns of physical, sexual, psychological, emotional, and/or economic abuse. Power and control are at the core of the problem. [Reprinted from New York State Office for the Prevention of Domestic Violence. Troy, New York, 1990. (Adapted with permission from Domestic Abuse Intervention Project, Duluth, Minnesota).]

The doctor finds that there are no retinal hemorrhages or internal signs of injury. The ecchymosis and injection are limited. The doctor, deciding that to treat only the external symptoms would be to overlook the underlying cause, returns to the issue of the origin of the box. The doctor hopes that during the course of the exam the patient's trust has been gained and that the patient will respond to the question now.

DR. BRADLEY: Ms. Marlowe, I have found that there is fortunately no extensive damage caused by your injury this time; however, if a similar incident happens again, I don't know if we would be as lucky. You said that a box hit you, and I am concerned about where it came from. Can you tell me where the box came from?

MS. MARLOWE: I was just sitting in my living room, and the box hit me. (Again, the patient seems hesitant. Although she had maintained eye contact with the doctor throughout the examination, suddenly she starts looking away. It is clear that there is something that concerns the patient about this question.)

DR. BRADLEY: In many cases, when I see a patient with a "black eye" like this, they tell me that a husband or someone they know caused the injury. Is it possible someone threw that box at you? (The doctor says this in a direct, but not accusing, tone.)

MS. MARLOWE: It . . . was . . . my husband. (The patient starts to cry.) He has been doing this for years. Sometimes it is even worse. I have three young children. I am afraid that he is going to start doing this to them.

Once the patient disclosed this, she started talking more. She said that her husband had also raped her repeatedly, and that she is afraid that he will do this to her daughters, too. Dr. Bradley followed the four-step plan (see p. 198) and provided the patient with phone numbers and contact people at a local women's shelter and counseling agency. She also offered ongoing, unconditional support and warmth. This was much more effective than treating only the "black eye."

Working with victims of domestic violence, and encouraging disclosures, can be difficult. Certain steps can enhance the clinician's ability to provide optimal intervention.

Strategies for Interaction

1. Use facilitative interviewing techniques and empathic responding to encourage disclosures.
2. If someone has accompanied the victim to the clinical examination, talk with each of them separately. Look for inconsistencies in the stories told by both individuals.
3. As in cases of suspected child abuse, look for multiple signs of injury, repeated episodes, and multiple stages of bruising to confirm your suspicions.
4. Ask the patient about the injuries. Give the patient an opportunity to explain how the injuries occurred:

Did someone cause these injuries?

Is there someone at home who threatens you, or harms you?

Does your spouse/partner ever threaten, harm, or strike you?

Does your partner ever hurt or harm your children?

Many patients who have similar signs tell me that someone they live with hits them, or hurts them. Could this be happening to you?

5. Educate the patient about local community services: counseling, legal, educational, and child-care services may be available.
6. Reassure the victim that she is not to blame for her battering. Validating the patient's experience, providing education, and expressing respect and support for the patient can be a successful start toward freedom from domestic violence.
7. The New York State Office for the Prevention of Domestic Violence suggests that health care professionals can benefit by "reframing" their idea of success in dealing with these cases. It is unrealistic to expect that a woman will just walk out and leave her partner after many years. Women often leave and return to their partner many times before they leave for good. Women may be hesitant to leave because of fear, embarrassment, religious beliefs, family pressures, lack of financial resources, inadequate housing and shelter, insufficient child-care services, and poor job training.

Four steps for successful interventions:

1. Identify signs of physical violence. The first step in handling abuse is properly identifying the physical signs.
2. Validate the patient's experience and feelings. Reassure the victim that her feelings of fear, isolation, confusion, anger, pain, and vulnerability are normal.
3. Advocate for the victim's safety and options. Inform the patient of local resources. These may include battered women's shelters, domestic violence hotlines, counseling and medical agencies, legal aid services, and neighborhood crisis centers.
4. Provide ongoing, unconditional support. Make sure that the victim knows that you are willing to be of assistance to her. Let her know that if she wants to speak to you further, she can call or return to see you.

ALCOHOLISM

Alcoholism has been recognized as one of the major public health concerns in the United States. The cost of alcoholism to society was estimated as $117 billion for a single year, including lost working days and medical costs (Goldman 1992). Approximately 20% of all males will experience clinically significant alcoholism at some point in their lives (Cohen-Cole 1991). A large proportion of all automobile fatalities are associated with alcohol use (Goldman 1992) and approximately one of every three arrests is associated with alcohol consumption (Coleman 1976). The life span of the average alcoholic individual is approximately 12 years shorter than the life span of the normal nonalcoholic individual (Coleman 1976).

Alcoholism has been considered to result from genetic and biochemical factors, sociocultural factors, and emotional pressures. Drinking is a widely socially accepted activity and many alcoholics justify their drinking as "normal" and refer to themselves as "social drinkers."

A common characteristic of alcoholics is denial. Denial makes it difficult to establish a pattern of alcohol use in many individuals. Patients frequently do not respond to direct questions about alcoholism or alcohol consumption. Alcoholics rarely admit or think that they drink too much, and when questioned they often deny use or abuse of alcohol. Many feel that they are still in control of their drinking.

Strategies for Interaction

1. Learn to identify the signs of alcohol abuse. The presence of alcohol on the patient's breath, slurred speech, and decreased motor control should alert the doctor to the possibility of alcoholism and indicate further inquiry about alcohol use.
2. Patients often evade direct questions about alcohol use. Questions such as "Have you been drinking more alcohol than you used to" are usually more conducive to responses than questions such as "Are you an alcoholic." Questions about alcohol consumption in the morning can be helpful. Most individuals who drink "socially" do not drink in the mornings. An individual who drinks in the morning, either to relieve a "hangover" from the night before or to help begin the day, may be an alcoholic.
3. The "CAGE" interview has been recommended as a useful technique in obtaining information about alcohol abuse (Ewing 1984). The four letters of CAGE form a mnemonic to assist the interviewer in remembering four key questions:

    Have you ever felt the need to cut down on your drinking?

    Do you ever get annoyed when people tell you to cut down on your drinking?

    Do you ever feel guilty about drinking too much?

    Do you ever need an eye-opener in the mornings?

4. Ask "how much do you drink" rather than "do you drink too much." The latter, qualitative question may produce a subjective answer. Individuals with a tolerance to alcohol may consume the equivalent of a liter or more of hard liquor per day (Goldman 1992). Friends or rela-

tives accompanying a patient may be helpful in providing information about an individual's drinking patterns.

5. Many of the patterns associated with alcoholism are also associated with drug abuse. Ask patients who abuse alcohol about their use of drugs.

6. Be attentive and responsive to the patient's affective messages.

7. To optimize responses from patients, start with general, broad, nonthreatening questions, and move to more specific questioning as information is elicited.

8. Be flexible and adaptive in your approach. If a patient does not appear to respond cooperatively to questions regarding alcohol consumption at the beginning of the examination, try to gather further information later during the examination, or at the end when clinical testing is completed. It may also be helpful to rephrase questions and ask for information in a less intimidating way.

9. Follow up when a pattern of alcoholism is identified. Be familiar with local referral sources and services that are available: alcoholism treatment programs, detoxification facilities, and rehabilitation units may be options; Alcoholics Anonymous, Al-Anon, and other organizations provide support and education for those who are ready to deal with an alcohol problem.

10. Referral to a general physician is advisable for further investigation on how alcohol use is affecting a patient's general medical status.

DRUG AND SUBSTANCE ABUSE

Like alcoholism, drug abuse and substance abuse have become major health concerns in the United States. Inappropriate use of drugs can result from:

1. Taking prescribed drugs in incorrect doses.
2. Taking drugs that have been prescribed for another individual.
3. Using an inappropriate combination of drugs.
4. Using illegal drugs.

Individuals may abuse drugs to deal with physical, social, psychological, and emotional problems. Drug abuse can interfere with a person's health and ability to function in occupational, avocational, and psychosocial activities. The World Health Organization defines addiction as "a behavioral pattern of drug use characterized by overwhelming involvement with the use of a drug, compulsive drug-seeking behavior, and a high tendency to relapse after withdrawal." The individual's life and behavior are controlled by the addiction.

Two types of dependence are associated with drug abuse: physical dependence and psychological dependence. Physical dependence can occur with a variety of psychoactive drugs. Psychoactive drugs include substances such as stimulants (e.g., amphetamines, "crack"), depressants (e.g., barbiturates), hallucinogens (e.g., LSD), opiates (e.g., codeine and opium), and marijuana. These drugs affect mental processes and have been widely misused. Many drugs produce a tolerance in which increasingly elevated amounts of a drug have to be utilized to produce the same results. Psychological dependence and motivation to continue to use a drug are also common with psychoactive drugs.

Like alcoholics, drug and substance abusers rarely present to the doctor to discuss their problem. Frequently, they deny any association with drug and substance abuse.

Strategies for Interaction

1. Start with general, nonthreatening questions. Work toward more specific information. Asking a direct question too early in the interview ("Do you have a problem with drug abuse?") may create a barrier to further inquiries on this topic. If the patient is evasive early in the interview, the doctor may find it helpful to ask further questions later in the course of the examination.

2. Adapt your approach. If initial inquiries about drug abuse are denied, try to obtain information on progressing levels. Ask initially about prescription medications (types, dosage, and frequency) and then about drugs that were not prescribed (types, dosage, and frequency), to delve into the area of drug abuse. The interviewer may then proceed to ask the patient, "Do you use any recreational drugs?" with corresponding follow-up questions.

3. Modify the "CAGE" mnemonic (see previous section, on alcoholism) to obtain relevant information on the use of drugs:

   Do you ever feel that you should cut down on your use of drugs?

   Do you ever get annoyed when people tell you to cut down on your use of drugs?

   Do you ever feel guilty about using drugs too often?

   Do you ever need an eye-opener of drugs in the mornings?

4. Look for ocular signs and manifestations of drug and substance abuse. Talc retinopathy, ptosis, nystagmus, diplopia, blurred vision, pupillary changes, and solar retinopathy are some of the ocular signs associated with drug and substance abuse (McLane and Carroll 1986).

5. Be familiar with and advise the patient of local referral sources and services that are available. Treatment programs, detoxification facilities, and rehabilitation units may be available. Self-help groups such as Narcotics Anonymous can be valuable in providing support and education for patients.
6. Referral to a general physician is helpful for further information on the effect of drug and substance abuse on a patient's general medical status.

STRATEGIES FOR WORKING WITH SPECIFIC PATIENT GROUPS

1. Recognize the challenges involved in working with patients from special groups to help identify useful strategies.
2. Identify realistic goals for patient management. Listen carefully to determine the patient's needs so your clinical management plans correspond with a patient's personal priorities and desires.
3. Develop an effective rapport with the patient's family members and caretakers to improve the quality of clinical encounters.
4. Many patients can benefit from local resources and agencies. Become familiar with services in your area, and inform patients of appropriate resources.
5. Remember the importance of interdisciplinary interactions. Sending reports and making referrals to general internists, psychologists, audiologists, and other health care professionals can improve the patient's overall clinical care.

QUESTIONS FOR THOUGHT

1. Provide four recommendations for interacting optimally with the following categories of patients:
   a. non-English-speaking patients,
   b. patients who abuse drugs, and
   c. hearing-impaired individuals.
2. Discuss the physical, physiological, sensory, and motor changes that occur with aging. How would you modify your examination sequence to optimize conditions for geriatric patients?
3. You are working with a patient with a low vision condition that has advanced recently. The patient is a 79-year-old female. You sense that she is depressed about this situation, and you are concerned about her level of distress. What can you do to help this patient?
4. You examine a 37-year-old male patient. On performing ophthalmoscopy, you see cotton wool spots. The patient had a complete physi-

cal examination two months ago, and you can rule out other causes; you are considering a possibility of HIV infection. What do you say to the patient, and how do you bring this topic up?
5. A 7-year-old child is brought to your office by her parents. There are bruises on both sides of the child's face. You look into the eyes and see retinal hemorrhages in both eyes. The mother says that the child fell on the way home from school yesterday. You suspect that the bruises may be signs of child abuse. What steps can you take to investigate your suspicions of child abuse?
6. A patient presents for a clinical examination. You smell alcohol, and suspect that the patient may abuse alcohol. What types of questions would you ask to determine whether this patient has a drinking problem? If you identify that the patient does abuse alcohol, how would you handle the situation?

REFERENCES

Attarian PJ. The Sexual History. In Levinson D, ed., A Guide to the Clinical Interview. Philadelphia: W.B. Saunders, 1987: 226–234.

Cohen-Cole SA. The Medical Interview: The Three-Function Approach. St. Louis: Mosby Year Book, 1991.

Cole RG. Considerations in Low Vision Prescribing. In Rosenthal BP, Cole RG, eds., Problems in Optometry—A Structured Approach to Low Vision Care, 3(3):416, 1991.

Coleman JC. Abnormal Psychology and Modern Life. Glenview, IL: Scott Foresman, 1976.

DiMatteo MR. The Psychology of Health, Illness, and Medical Care. Pacific Grove, CA: Brooks/Cole, 1991.

Ewing JA. Detecting alcoholism: The CAGE questionnaire. Journal of the American Medical Association 252:1905, 1984.

Fleisher GR, Ludwig S. Textbook of Pediatric Emergency Medicine. Baltimore: Williams & Wilkins, 1988.

Freeman P. Initiating successful low vision care. Practical Optometry 2(2):56–58, 1991.

Freeman PB, Jose RT. The Art and Practice of Low Vision. Boston: Butterworth-Heinemann, 1991.

Goldman HH. Review of General Psychiatry. Norwalk, CT: Appleton & Lange, 1992.

Holmes TH, Rahe RH. The social readjustment rating scale. Journal of Psychosomatic Research 11:213–218, 1967.

Kessler DB, Hyden P. Clinical Symposia: Physical, Sexual, and Emotional Abuse of Children. Summit, NJ: Ciba-Geigy, 1991.

Lovie-Kitchin JE, Bowman KJ. Senile Macular Degeneration—Management and Rehabilitation. Boston: Butterworth, 1985.

McLane NJ, Carroll DM. Ocular manifestations of drug abuse. Survey of Ophthalmology 30(5):298–313, 1986.

Mehr EB, Fried AN. Low Vision Care. Boston: Butterworth-Heinemann, 1975.

New York State Office for the Prevention of Domestic Violence. Domestic Violence Data Sheet. 200 Broadway, Third Floor, Troy, NY 12180, 1990.

Optometric Gerontology: A Resource Manual. Association of Schools and Colleges of Optometry, 6110 Executive Boulevard, Suite 514, Rockville, MD 20852, 1989.

Shindell S. Psychological sequelae to diabetic retinopathy. Journal of the American Optometric Association 59(11):870–874, 1988.

Shute RH. Psychology in Vision Care. Oxford: Butterworth-Heinemann, 1991.

Smith SK. Child abuse and neglect: A diagnostic guide for the optometrist. Journal of the American Optometric Association 59(10):760–766, 1988.

Weinman J. An Outline of Psychology as Applied to Medicine. Bristol: Wright, 1987.

Weinstein BE. Geriatric hearing loss: Myths, realities, resources for physicians. Geriatrics 44(4):42–58, 1989.

Weinstein BE. Auditory testing and rehabilitation of the hearing impaired. In Lubinski R, ed., Dementia: Clinical Implications and Research. Philadelphia: Dexter Publications, 1990.

Ventry I, Weinstein BE. Identification of elderly people with hearing problems. American Speech-Language-Hearing Association (ASHA) July:37–42, 1983.

ADDITIONAL READINGS

Bilingual Medical Interview I. Boston Department of Health & Hospitals, 818 Harrison Avenue, Boston, MA 02118.

Bilingual Medical Interview II: The Geriatric Interview. Boston Department of Health & Hospitals, 818 Harrison Avenue, Boston, MA 02118.

Birren JE, Schaie KW. Handbook of the Psychology of Aging. San Diego: Academic Press, 1990.

Chez RA. Physician's guide: Evaluation of the abused woman. Medical Aspects of Human Sexuality 8:32–36, 1989.

Ham RJ, Sloane PD. Primary Care Geriatrics: A Case-Based Approach. St. Louis: Mosby Year Book, 1992.

Randall T. Domestic violence calls for more than treating injuries. Journal of the American Medical Association 264(8):939–940, 1990.

Thorn F, Thorn S, Ziemian DM. TV captions are difficult to read with small amounts of blur. NEWENCO Research Series 1991. The New England College of Optometry, 424 Beacon Street, Boston, MA 02115.

Wood TE. Communicating with hearing-impaired individuals. Journal of the American Optometric Association 58(1):62–65, 1987.

14

Handling Difficult Patient Encounters

"Difficult" patients present with communication challenges. Understanding the dynamics of the communication can sometimes be the key to handling the situation optimally.

When approaching "difficult" patients, it is always helpful to consider the patient's motivation and what the doctor can do to improve the situation. Many doctors try to ignore a patient's negative emotions and just concentrate on the clinical tasks. Although this may appear to be a very professional attitude, it often does not meet the patient's needs. When patients present with an affective, emotional expression, acknowledging their comments can allow the patient to move on. Sometimes just saying "I see that you are angry; how can I help you?" or "I can tell that you are very nervous; can I do anything to make you more comfortable?" can meet the patient's needs. Doctors who counter a patient's affective comments with factual responses will often be ineffective. Like psychiatric patients, "difficult" patients are often labeled with pejorative terms. "Grief" case, nuts, pain in the neck (PITN), and crazy are just a few examples. Doctors should recognize that negative terms and attitudes can impact on the quality of care (Groves 1978). Although these patients present with challenging interpersonal styles, they are entitled to good, competent, compassionate health care.

In this chapter, a set of "difficult" patient types will be discussed, and recommendations for working with each of them will be given. These recommendations are meant as suggestions as to how one may go about handling a situation. Additional strategies for working with difficult people have been discussed (Alessandra and O'Connor 1990; Bramson 1981; Keating 1984; Groves 1978; Levinson 1987; Cohen-Cole 1991; Muchnick and Nyman 1992). Different styles and techniques may be applied and adapted on an individual basis. The reader is invited to come up with other approaches that may work optimally for him or her.

"SILENT" PATIENT

It is usually very difficult to get a good case history from very quiet patients who are often intimidated by open-ended questions. Closed-ended questions often present a more manageable way for these patients to provide information. Patients are sometimes quiet because they are nervous, uncomfortable, tired, or afraid. Understanding the patient's reason for silence will help the doctor choose an appropriate approach to communication.

Strategies for Interaction

1. Try closed-ended questions during the case history, rather than open-ended ones, to try to get the patient to talk.
2. Use "laundry list" questions to encourage patients to respond.
3. Use facilitative questions and behaviors (Chapters 2 and 3) to get the patient to continue speaking (e.g., "Tell me more about that" or "Keep going").
4. Ask patients if there is anything you can do to make them more comfortable.
5. If patients are very reticent and reserved in response to clinical questions, it is sometimes helpful to get them to talk about topics that are more familiar to them. Common topics are a patient's occupation, holiday plans, or leisure activities. Once patients start to talk about something that interests them, it is often easier to get them to talk about the information you need.
6. Provide reassurance and create a safe and supportive environment.

> DR. MAZUR: What brings you in today? (The doctor starts the case history with a general, open-ended question.)
>
> MR. LEFF: Uh . . . an eye exam.
>
> DR. MAZUR: Oh, so you need an eye examination today. Tell me, what types of problems have you been experiencing? (Again, the doctor tries a broad, open-ended question.)
>
> MR. LEFF: Uh . . . well, . . . not too many problems. (At this point, the doctor realizes that there is difficulty getting answers with open-ended questions and decides to change strategy and ask more constricted, closed-ended questions.)
>
> DR. MAZUR: Does your vision ever get blurry at distance?

MR. LEFF: No.

DR. MAZUR: How about at near? Any blurry vision at near?

MR. LEFF: Sometimes.

DR. MAZUR: How long have you noticed your vision at near is blurry?

MR. LEFF: Um, . . . well, . . . (thinking). (Seeing that the patient is having trouble answering this, Dr. Mazur makes use of a laundry list question.)

DR. MAZUR: Is it closer to a week, or a month, or six months? Or some other length of time?

MR. LEFF: I guess about a month. It gets real blurry sometimes.

DR. MAZUR: How long do you have to be reading for your vision to get blurry? (The doctor takes a chance at this point that the patient may be able to respond without the laundry list and asks a broader question.)

MR. LEFF: About half an hour. I can read for a few minutes, but then it gets really blurry. And my eyes start to feel really uncomfortable. (The patient has begun to express himself more, and broader questions are now a viable option.)

DR. MAZUR: Tell me about the discomfort. What does it feel like? (The doctor continues the interview; the patient is more talkative at this point.)

This interaction used a broad–narrow–broad approach (see Chapter 2). The doctor started with broad questions, as was routinely done. When the patient did not respond well, the doctor went to narrower questions. Then, once the patient was talking, the doctor was able to move to more open-ended inquiries.

"OVERTALKATIVE" OR RAMBLING PATIENT

The goal with overly talkative or rambling patients is to try to keep them focused on the examination and on the details that are needed for a particular situation. The doctor should always consider other factors that may be contributing to the patient's behavior, such as nervousness, stress, or the need to control the situation. A patient who is not normally verbose may become overly talkative when nervous. Making the patient more comfortable and relaxed may help control the reaction. Rambling patients tend to digress from one topic to another. To keep this encounter under control, focus your questions on the examination.

Strategies for Interaction

1. Ask direct, closed-ended questions; avoid vague, open-ended questions.

2. Learn to cut the patient off politely, when necessary, to bring the discussion back to the examination.
3. If patients appear concerned about their views not being considered in the decision-making phase, it is best to assure them in advance of your intention to include their wishes in your plan.

DR. SHAPIRO: What brings you in today, Ms. Brand?

MS. BRAND: I had trouble seeing the movie when I was on a plane recently, and I realized that I better have my glasses checked. I travel a lot, and it's not easy for me to take the time to set up an appointment. Anyway, the flight was delayed, and I got to my business meeting about an hour late. It was a rough day for me.

DR. SHAPIRO: Ms. Brand, you mention that you noticed that you had trouble seeing the movie on the plane. Have you noticed your vision blurry on any other occasions? (The doctor returns the conversation to the topic of her vision, and proceeds with the next question. The brief interaction so far has not yet established that she is an "overly talkative" patient, and in this case the doctor chooses to go with an open-ended question.)

MS. BRAND: Sometimes I notice that when I'm driving, the signs in the distance are hard to see until I get closer. But it seemed worse on the plane. It's probably because that was such a difficult day, anyway. I woke up late that morning, and I almost missed that flight. I got there about 5 minutes before they finished boarding all of the passengers. (The patient takes the liberty in answering the doctor's previous open-ended question with detail; the doctor has gotten some useful information about the patient's vision when she drives, but now realizes that it is appropriate to cut her off.)

DR. SHAPIRO: Is your vision ever blurry at near? (The doctor asks a closed-ended question, hoping to get a more limited answer.)

MS. BRAND: No, I can read fine, even for hours without a problem. It's the distance that I'm interested in. Like on that plane, I really would have liked to see that movie. (Even with closed-ended questions, "overly talkative" patients may start to ramble, but the doctor can usually get the required information at the beginning of the response. This doctor continues to ask closed-ended questions, and cuts the patient off politely when necessary.)

DR. PENN: Ms. Rothman, how can I help you today? (The doctor starts off all case histories with an open-ended question, and is not yet aware that this is a "rambling" patient.)

MS. ROTHMAN: I figured it was time for an eye examination. I've been busy moving and visiting relatives and I kept forgetting to call for an appointment. I went to Chicago last month and visited my niece and her family, and I stayed there two weeks. They had a big snow storm there, but it finally started to get a little warmer. (The doctor gets some sense that this may be a rambling patient, and redirects the patient's attention back to the examination, cutting in with the next comment when the patient pauses.)

DR. PENN: Was there any particular problem or concern that led you to make the appointment, or are you just here for a general examination? (This question is directed back to the examination, but is still fairly general and open-ended.)

MS. ROTHMAN: I just figured it was time for a general examination. I haven't really thought about whether I have any problems because I have been so busy. I've had a lot of deadlines at work and I am writing a report that is due next week. I have a new client whom I met on a trip to Hawaii, and I am preparing a report for her. We had such a great time in Hawaii. The weather was fantastic, and the hotel where we stayed was gorgeous. (By this point, the doctor's suspicion that this patient is a "rambler" is confirmed.)

DR. PENN: Ms. Rothman, when you are working on the reports at work, is your vision always clear, or do you experience any problems seeing things close up? (The doctor brings the discussion back to the eye examination, and asks a specific question about the patient's vision in a particular task.)

It is important to listen to a patient's concerns, and to let the patient express problems; however, when a patient's responses are excessive, the doctor should realize that this serves neither the patient's needs nor those of the other patients in the doctor's practice. Allowing the patient to continue to go on can put the doctor significantly behind schedule and other patients may be kept waiting. Using time ineffectively does not benefit the patient or the doctor.

"NERVOUS" PATIENT

Patients who are nervous are usually concerned about some aspect of the examination. They may be afraid that a clinical procedure will be uncomfortable or painful or they may be concerned that the doctor will find something wrong with them. Often, by letting patients know that you have observed that they are apprehensive or nervous, and by asking if there is anything that you can do to make them more comfortable, the patients become more relaxed. Demonstrating a caring, compassionate attitude can assist the doctor in helping this type of patient.

Strategies for Interaction

1. Try to identify what is making the patient nervous. Show interest in the patient's concern. Make sure patients know that you understand what is on their mind.
2. Ask if there is anything you can do to make the patient more comfortable.

3. Look for hidden agendas. Often, by identifying concerns that the patient has *not* expressed, the doctor can pinpoint the source of the patient's discomfort.
4. Create a safe and supportive environment for the patient, and provide reassurance.

> Mr. Reynolds is a 79-year-old male with cataracts, presenting to the eye doctor for a general examination. His facial expression is very serious, his body posture is very tense, and his eye contact is very limited. He is tapping his feet on the floor, and squeezing his hands on the arms of the examination chair.
>
> DR. MEREDITH: Mr. Reynolds, you seem to be a little nervous today. Is there anything I can do to make you feel more comfortable?
>
> MR. REYNOLDS: Well, I guess I'm sort of worried about my vision. The doctor last year said that I have cataracts. Some of my friends have had cataract surgery recently. I'm worried that I may need to have cataract surgery. I have a heart condition, and I'm afraid that this would be a problem for surgery.
>
> DR. MEREDITH: I understand that you're worried about the cataracts and the possible need for surgery. (The doctor paraphrases the patient's concern.) I'm going to check you very carefully today. Many people with cataracts do *not* need surgery, so it's possible that you may not need surgery at all at this point. If you do, we will check with your cardiologist to make sure that you are able to have surgery. I can assure you that we're not going to rush into anything. I'll examine you and tell you what I find. Then, we can discuss all the options. I'm going to work together *with you* to find a solution that makes you feel comfortable. Do you feel a little better about going through the examination now?

This example emphasizes the need to look for hidden agendas with "nervous" patients. By identifying the hidden agenda, and addressing the patient's concerns, the doctor can make the patient more prepared to focus on the details of the examination.

"ANGRY" PATIENT

This type of situation comprises one of the most challenging categories of "difficult" patients. It is often difficult to elicit information from these patients because of the strong emotional overtones. They may respond with anger and hostility during both the case history and the examination sequence. It is often futile to try to continue the clinical tasks and objectives without addressing the anger. Patients who are responding emotionally often need their affective level acknowledged *before* they are able to go on. Although the doctor may not be able to control how a patient presents to the office, the doctor can control his or her response to the situation. Effective doctors learn to handle these situations with positive strategies.

Strategies for Interaction

1. Consider using a three-step plan when working with these patients:
   a. Validate the emotional response of patients to show that you respect their feelings and understand their viewpoint. Validating the patient's response does not mean that you agree with the patient's reason for being angry. ("I can see you are upset about this situation.")
   b. Address the patient's problem. Say something to show that you understand the patient's complaint. ("I apologize for keeping you waiting so long.")
   c. Tell the patient what you are going to do about the problem. ("You have my undivided attention at this point, and I want to help you in any way I can.")
2. Always treat the patient with respect. Remember that even if you do not agree with the patient about a concern, that problem is probably very real to the patient.
3. Consider your potential response to an angry patient. Although it is a natural temptation to respond defensively or with anger, the doctor should realize that this reaction rarely serves a positive function. More than likely, it "fuels the fire" and makes the patient even angrier.
4. Try to understand *why* the patient is angry (Table 14.1). Some of these reasons may be legitimate (e.g., the patient was taken an hour late for the examination), and some may be considered totally unfounded (e.g.,

Table 14.1 Reasons why patients may become angry in the clinical environment

The patient may have arrived for the appointment on time and had to wait a long time to see the doctor.

The patient may be frustrated about the long waiting period for an appointment.

The patient may be concerned about being able to pay the doctor's fees.

The doctor may remind the patient of someone who made the patient angry previously, and the patient may demonstrate a "transference" toward the doctor.

The patient may have had frustrating experiences with the health care system previously and may be venting this frustration toward the current doctor.

The patient may have had a difficult day at the office and may be releasing this anger at the time of the clinical appointment.

The patient may be nervous or uncomfortable and may be expressing any of a range of feelings in the form of anger.

The doctor, or a member of the staff, may have said something to the patient that was misinterpreted and that upset the patient, even if the comment was not meant in the way that it was interpreted.

The doctor, or a member of the staff, may have said something that justifiably resulted in the patient's anger.

the doctor and staff feel that the patient walked into the office angry, and nothing in the office provoked the anger). Whether the reason is legitimate or not, the doctor should remember that from the *patient's* viewpoint, the anger is justified.

MS. BARROWS: I can't believe it. I have waited almost two weeks for these contact lenses. Now I've put them on and you tell me that the prescription needs to be changed. This has taken so long.

DR. HONG: I can see that you are upset, Ms. Barrows. (Acknowledges patient's anger.) I know that you have waited a long time, and I apologize for the wait. Your contact lenses are custom lenses, and as we explained to you when you ordered them, it usually takes a little longer to get custom lenses. I'm sorry that you had to wait. (Addresses the patient's problem.) I'm going to let you use these lenses as a "loaner" and I'm going to arrange for the *fastest* way to get your new lenses delivered. That way you'll have them as soon as possible. (Tells the patient what is going to be done about the problem.)

DR. ARTHUR: I notice that you appear a little angry or nervous, Ms. Rogers. Is there anything that I can do to help make this a more pleasant experience for you? (The doctor acknowledges the patient's behavior somewhat indirectly, and in a nonthreatening tone.)

MS. ROGERS: Well, I've been sitting in your waiting room for over an hour, waiting to be taken, and now you're just asking me questions, and not even looking at my broken glasses.

DR. ARTHUR: I can understand how waiting can be frustrating. I'm sorry that you had to wait. We are running a little behind schedule this afternoon. We usually try to stick as close to the schedule as possible, but sometimes something unexpected occurs. I'm sorry for the wait—I know that waiting can be disturbing. (The doctor addresses the patient's problem.) Now, let me take a look at your glasses. I'm very interested in looking at your broken glasses so I can see how to help you. (The doctor shows empathy for the patient's frustration, apologizes that the patient was kept waiting, expresses interest in the patient's concern—the broken glasses—and attends to her problem.) Tell me about what happened to your glasses.

MS. ROGERS: I broke my frame two weeks ago, and I'm having a very difficult time reading my notes without my glasses. (The patient responds to the doctor's inquiry about her chief complaint, and she now provides the necessary information for the doctor to start the examination.)

"MALINGERING" PATIENT

Malingerers are individuals who are purposely trying to feign an illness or medical problem. Patients sometimes malinger to get attention or to acquire financial gain. If it is possible to establish the reason for malingering, the doctor can take steps to help the patient deal with the underlying problem. If a teenager is under excessive stress, or if an adult is having psychological problems, recommending appropriate counseling is indicated. When dealing with a suspected malingerer, it is important to make sure that other problems have not been overlooked.

Strategies for Interaction

1. Try to assess the patient's motivation by looking for inconsistencies in the patient's report of signs, symptoms, and problems or using clinical methods specifically designed for malingerers (e.g., spiral visual fields, using a +0.12 lens to see if it makes a significant difference in the patient's visual acuity).
2. Don't label a patient as a "malingerer" unless you are certain that the problems described are not attributable to clinical causes.
3. When indicated, proper referrals to mental health professionals (e.g., psychologists, psychiatrists, social workers) are in order (see Chapters 10 and 15).
4. Learn to distinguish the "malingerer" from the "hysterical" patient who has an underlying psychological problem characterized by unconscious lying. Listening carefully to the patient's report of the problems and using some of the clinical techniques to identify malingerers is helpful. Differentiating these situations is an important step in helping the patient.

"KNOW-IT-ALL" PATIENT

"Know-it-all" patients can be particularly disturbing to doctors because they convey a lack of confidence in the doctor's judgment. They may come in and tell the doctor what tests need to be done and what therapeutic steps need to be taken. The "know-it-all" patient who disagrees with the doctor will not hesitate to say so.

Some "know-it-all" patients are anxious and nervous. They try to appear knowledgeable to get doctors to practice at their best. Some may have had negative experiences with the health care delivery system in the past, and are trying to prevent such errors from occurring in the future. Others may try to obtain more attention from their doctors. It is often helpful to reassure patients of your interest in their problems. However, the doctor should recognize that excessive attention may reinforce a patient's need for attention.

Strategies for Interaction

1. Consider the motivation for the patient's attitude and tailor your reaction appropriately. Ask patients how they became so informed in a

particular area or how they gained so much experience on a specific issue. Learn to differentiate the patient who is anxious or nervous from the one who has had previous negative experiences with health care.

2. Praise the patient's knowledge and understanding (if this is appropriate) and efforts to understand the clinical status. Assure patients that you will invite their involvement and participation when management plans are determined.
3. Express empathy for previous difficulties with the health care delivery system if appropriate and state your sincere interest and dedication to the patient.
4. Discussing your credentials and experience in a specialty area can help build patient confidence.
5. Reassure the patient of your dedication, competence, and attention.

> Ms. Walters, I can understand that you had some problems with these symptoms previously. I want you to know that I am very interested in your problem and that I can understand your concern. I also want you to be reassured that I will do my best to find out what is bothering you. After I complete my tests, I will explain all of my findings, and we can work together to decide what will be best for you. (Patients in this category often want to know that they will be able to participate in the decision-making process. Reassurance often helps allay their concern. Sometimes it is helpful to mention the doctor's credentials and competence.)
>
> Ms. Walters, I want you to know that I have been in this practice for 15 years, and I have treated many patients with your problem. I'll be happy to examine you, and when I am finished we can work together to decide what treatment will be best for you.

"SEDUCTIVE" PATIENT

Patients sometimes exhibit sexually seductive behaviors toward their doctors. They may dress seductively, touch the doctor, display flirtatious behaviors, offer intimate details about themselves that are unrelated to the clinical care, or ask questions about the doctor's personal life.

Sexual interest may result when patients are attracted to the power and esteem of the doctor. This behavior may be the result of the transference of attitudes and feelings from other relationships to the doctor. (Transference and its management are discussed in Chapter 6, pp. 82–84.) It is important for the doctor to try to understand the patient's motivation and to realize that the basis for the patient's behavior is not inherent in the doctor.

Patients may look to their doctors for support, compassion, and intimacy. Although patients may not really be interested in having an actual physical encounter with the doctor, the sexual behavior may make them feel closer to and more intimate with the doctor; ironically, the caring relationship of the doctor–patient rapport may intensify the patient's behavior.

The doctor should remember that it is considered unethical to take advantage of the patient's seductive behavior. It is essential for the doctor to know how to handle this situation appropriately.

Strategies for Interaction

1. Initially, try to ignore the seductive behavior of the patient and continue with the clinical examination in a professional manner. When patients notice that the doctor is not responding as they wish, patients often realize that the behaviors are not desired and will desist. Sometimes reassuring patients of your professional interest in them, and discouraging seductive comments, is enough to stop the inappropriate actions.
2. If the behaviors continue, the doctor must become more direct. By speaking nonjudgmentally, and in a way that does not embarrass the patient, the doctor should be able to maintain a therapeutic relationship with the patient.
3. It may be helpful to have an office technician sit in on the examination to assist with procedures. Having someone else in the room should discourage inappropriate comments. If questions arise later about the doctor's conduct, the assistant can serve as a witness to confirm that the doctor has acted in a professional manner.

Ms. Arpen is a 41-year-old female, presenting to the eye doctor for a general examination. She frequently interacts in a very personal manner with the doctor. When this occurs, he politely tries to return the conversation back to the examination.

The doctor demonstrates good listening skills and gives the patient ample opportunity to express her concerns. He maintains a pleasant disposition, but makes sure that the interaction retains a professional tone. When he needs to set firm limits, he makes sure that his nonverbal cues match his more serious tone.

DR. VERGOS: Good morning. What brings you in today, Ms. Arpen?

MS. ARPEN: Well, it's always good to see you. That's a good reason, isn't it? (Smiling and spoken in a flirtatious tone.)

DR. VERGOS: Thank you. I'm always glad to take care of my patients. (Ignoring her previous tone, and trying to return to the examination.) Have you had any problems with your vision recently?

MS. ARPEN: Have I ever! My vision at near is going downhill. I can be going through the mail, and the print on the page just starts to blend together. (Pausing.) Do you think it's my age? Do you think I look OK?

DR. VERGOS: You look fine, Ms. Arpen (neutral tone). Now I need to ask you some other questions about your vision. How is your distance vision?

MS. ARPEN: Oh, that's just fine. I never have a problem with that. I can see lots of details when I look around. Like your suit. You look so good in that suit.

DR. VERGOS: Thank you. (The doctor responds in a neutral tone, trying to discourage the personal comments. Then he quickly returns to the examination.) Ms. Arpen, when you start to read, how long does it take for your vision to get blurry?

MS. ARPEN: Oh, it can be just a few minutes, and I feel like my eyes are going around in my head. It's really annoying. (Pause.) I'm glad I came back to you. I always feel comfortable when I'm with you.

DR. VERGOS: Have you noticed any other changes?

MS. ARPEN: At my age, everything is starting to go. (She laughs.) Even my hair is starting to turn gray. (She laughs again.) Do you have any gray hair? (Staring at the doctor.) I don't think I see any. You look so attractive.

DR. VERGOS: (The doctor realizes that his previous approach has not worked, and that he must set firm limits.) Ms. Arpen, we really must keep our conversation on your examination. I am flattered by your compliments, but we really must keep a professional relationship. I would really appreciate it if we could keep our comments related to the exam. You are a very important patient in our office, and I would like to help solve your vision problems. (Pause.) So tell me, are you seeing clearly at distance? (This patient has a true clinical concern resulting from presbyopia. By interacting with the patient respectfully and effectively, the doctor has been able to address her problems and maintain a therapeutic relationship.)

Mr. Jackson is a 42-year-old patient who presents to Dr. Kane's office for the first time. He lives in the local community but has not formally met the doctor.

DR. KANE: What brings you in for an eye examination today, Mr. Jackson?

MR. JACKSON: I just figured it was time to get my eyes checked. It's been about three years since my last exam, and I figured that's a pretty long time. I also thought it would be a good excuse to stop in and see you. (During the case history the patient displays some flirtatious behavior in comments, tone, and eye contact with the doctor. The doctor tries to discourage his behavior by ignoring the flirtation. Toward the end of the case history, his comments become more direct.)

MR. JACKSON: You know, you're asking so many questions about me. Don't I get to ask some questions about you? (Smiling.) I'd really like to know a little more about you (suggestive tone).

DR. KANE: (The doctor realizes at this point that she must become more direct with the patient.) Mr. Jackson, we really must maintain a professional relationship. I'd appreciate it if you could keep your comments on the examination so I can help you.

MR. JACKSON: That's OK with me. We can talk about the examination. OK, I'll answer your questions about my eyes. (The patient does respond to the doctor's request at this point, and for a while he limits his responses to clinical information. During the examination, he starts making suggestive comments again, and at one point he makes the following remark.) When are you going to get to the test where you look in my eyes? You can look in my eyes anytime. (This is of great concern to the doctor because she feels that the patient's behavior is inappropriate. She is also greatly concerned that he will misinterpret a clinical examination [ophthalmoscopy]. Before she continues, she feels that she must get a commitment from the patient that the interaction will remain professional, and that he understands that any suggestive behaviors must stop.)

DR. KANE: Mr. Jackson, I really can't go on unless I am sure that you realize that our discussion must only continue on a professional basis. It makes me very uncomfortable when you make some of your comments. I'd really like to help you with your eyes, but I need to know that we understand the reason for our meeting today.

MR. JACKSON: Well, I guess I have been making some comments. If it makes you uncomfortable, I'll stop them.

DR. KANE: I really appreciate that, Mr. Jackson. I want to assure you that my intent is to give you the best clinical care. I also want to make sure that you understand that when I do ophthalmoscopy, which is when I look in your eyes, that I am doing it solely as a clinical procedure.

MR. JACKSON: Yes, I do realize that. I have heard many comments on what a good doctor you are. (The rest of the examination proceeds uneventfully, and Dr. Kane has successfully established and maintained a professional relationship without making the patient feel uncomfortable.)

"GRIEF" PATIENT

The "grief" patient is a chronic complainer who finds fault with everything and constantly expresses dissatisfaction. As with the angry patient, the grief patient may evoke anger and frustration in the doctor or office staff. This response is counterproductive and may fuel the patient's emotional response. By validating a patient's dissatisfaction and expressing empathy, the doctor may be perceived as a more sensitive, understanding individual than previous caretakers.

DOCTOR: I can see why it would upset you that your previous doctor sent you an incorrect bill. I can assure you that the paperwork and care in our office are accurate, and we will do all we can to satisfy you.

Sometimes, no matter how hard the doctor and staff try to make a patient happy, the patient will find something to complain about. Doctors usually strive to have patients who are happy with their care, and who express satisfaction. Looking for approval from a "grief" patient is sometimes an unrealistic expectation. It can be suggested that if a "grief" patient *does not* find something to complain about, that this should be seen as a success.

Strategies for Interaction

1. Empathize with patients for their concerns, and try to find solutions to the problems when possible.
2. Set realistic goals. The grief patient is not likely to turn from excessive complainer to enthusiastic supporter overnight. Often, the best you can hope for is a neutral response.

DR. ORBER: What brings you in today, Mr. Johnson?

MR. JOHNSON: I wanted to try a new eye doctor because my last eye doctor always kept me waiting, and the one before that always seemed to rush me through the exam. The doctor in my old neighborhood never seemed very interested in my problems, just like my latest physician. (The patient expresses a consistent pattern of complaints; they may be legitimate complaints, or the doctor may suspect this as a "grief" patient.)

DR. ORBER: I can understand your discomfort with those situations. I can assure you that we are interested in any of your concerns here, and that we try to take our patients promptly. (The doctor expresses empathy with the patient's previous dissatisfaction, and conveys concern toward the patient's complaints; these are valuable steps in building good doctor–patient rapport with "grief" patients.)

The patient in the following case called the office by phone and insisted on speaking to the doctor about his complaint.

DR. STARR: Mr. Robertson, I heard that you called our office and that you were displeased with your glasses. What seems to be the problem?

MR. ROBERTSON: First, they gave me the glasses and they were too loose. Then they gave me the glasses and they were hurting me behind my ear. Then they gave me a hard case for my frames, but I don't like carrying around hard cases.

DR. STARR: Mr. Robertson, we'd be happy to readjust your frames for you. Please come into our office, and I would be happy to readjust your frames. When you come in, I'll be happy to replace your case with a soft case that you may find easier to carry around.

When the patient comes in to have the frames adjusted and exchange the case, the following discussion ensues:

DR. STARR: How do your glasses feel now, Mr. Robertson?

MR. ROBERTSON: They're OK, I guess. They're not too bad now. ("Grief" patients characteristically don't express satisfaction with something, so no complaint can actually be seen as a success.)

DR. STARR: I understand that you have picked out a different case to hold your glasses. Is this case what you had in mind?

MR. ROBERTSON: I guess it's better.

DR. STARR: That's great. Please feel free to let us know if you need the frames readjusted, or if there is anything else that we can do to help you. (The doctor reexpresses the commitment to satisfy the patient; this may be reassuring to the "grief" patient, although the patient may not verbally express reassurance.)

"EVASIVE" PATIENT

The "evasive" patient gives an impression of withholding information from the doctor. Consider *why* the patient may want to withhold information from you. If patients do not trust the doctor, they may not want to reveal personal information. If this is the case, the doctor needs to be presented as a more caring, supportive, trustworthy individual. Sometimes it is helpful to reassure the patient that it is important for doctors to gather a lot of information so they can make appropriate decisions. It is also helpful to reassure patients that their records are confidential.

Drug addicts, alcoholics, and victims of domestic violence sometimes try to conceal specific information. Asking questions in different forms, and at different times during the examination, can be helpful. It is particularly important to phrase questions in a nonthreatening style.

Strategies for Interaction

1. Consider what motivates the patient. Is there a lack of trust, or is the patient purposefully concealing information?
2. Try to build trust with the patient. Reassure patients of your support, concern, and interest in their needs.
3. When patients appear to be holding back information, it may be helpful to explain why you are asking a particular question. Explicitly assuring the individual of patient confidentiality can also be helpful.
4. Ask questions in different ways. If patients won't answer a question in one form, they may answer it in another. Use facilitative statements and questions to try to get the patient to continue speaking.
5. Move from broad, open-ended questions to narrow, specific questions as the patient becomes more comfortable in the environment.
6. Try to avoid language and tones that may appear threatening or antagonistic.
7. If you believe a patient abuses alcohol or drugs, try using some of the questions from the CAGE interview (see Chapter 13, pp. 198–200) to help obtain responses. Direct questions may sound accusatory.

8. When other techniques do not help, confronting statements and questions (Chapter 2) may help to accomplish the doctor's objectives.

DOCTOR: Ms. Pearlstone, you seem to be very apprehensive in discussing your general health. For me to help you optimally, I need to know about any medical problems that you may be having. (The doctor acknowledges the patient's apprehension, and expresses need for the information.)

PATIENT: I just don't like talking about my health with anybody. You never know who's going to find out about your personal information. (In response to the doctor's query, the patient expresses concern about whether details about her health will go beyond the doctor's office.)

DOCTOR: I can assure you that the records in our office are *completely* confidential, and that no one else has access to our records. You can be sure that I will not discuss any details about your health and medical status with anyone else. You are welcome to discuss any other concerns that you have with me, but I must also ask that you share any information about your health so that I can help you optimally. (The doctor reassures the patient that her clinical information is confidential and will not be discussed with anyone else, and asks her again to provide the necessary information.)

PATIENT: Well, the one thing on my mind is that I just had a blood test recently (hesitantly), and they found that I am HIV-positive. I don't know if that affects my eyes at all, and I am really concerned about that test result. (By hearing the doctor's reassurance about the confidentiality of the records, the patient discusses the problem that initially caused her to be evasive.)

DOCTOR: That must be a very difficult situation for you. (Showing empathy.) It's good that you told me about that because there are a number of things that I will do to try to help you. (The doctor reinforces the patient's decision to disclose, and provides relevant information to the patient.)

DR. LEE: Mr. Frampton, how is your general health?

MR. FRAMPTON: It's not too bad lately. (The patient responds with a brief, vague answer.)

DR. LEE: Do you have any particular problems with your general health? (The doctor perceives that the patient is somewhat evasive and aloof, and resorts to a more direct question.)

MR. FRAMPTON: Nothing that has to do with my eyes.

DR. LEE: It's very important that patients tell me when they have problems with their health. There are many medical problems that are associated with the eyes, and people are not always aware of that. For example, there are eye signs associated with hypertension and diabetes, and it's important to monitor the vision of these patients. If you have any problems with your health, I hope that you will feel comfortable to discuss them with me. (The doctor explains the reason for needing the information, and encourages the patient to disclose what is on his mind.)

MR. FRAMPTON: Well, they found a tumor on my lung last month, and I'm being treated for lung cancer. (Hesitantly.) Doctor, I know that my sister is a patient of yours. I haven't told the family yet, and I really wouldn't want her to know anything about this now.

DR. LEE: Mr. Frampton, you can be absolutely assured that I will not discuss this with anyone else without your permission. I can understand your desire for privacy, and your interest in discussing this with your family when you are ready. My concern is that you are getting the care that you need, so I am going to ask you a few questions about your treatment. If you wish, I would be happy to send a report to your physician after today's examination to provide information about your eye health, but other than that, I would not discuss your situation with anyone.

MR. FRAMPTON: Yes, I think that would be a good idea. My physician asked a lot of questions about me, and would probably find a report helpful.

"CONFUSED/FORGETFUL" OR "POOR HISTORIAN" PATIENT

Conducting a case history on this type of patient can be very challenging. Patients may have a difficult time responding because they are poorly focused on the questions or unsure of their answers. Provide reassurance and allow patients sufficient time to respond to questions. If "poor historians" are unable to answer a question, allow them to maintain their dignity and move to the next stage of the interview.

Strategies for Interaction

1. Provide additional time for the patient to think about answers to your questions.
2. Encourage the patient to respond and provide reassurance when answers are given.
3. Assure the patient that there are no "right" or "wrong" answers. Reinforce that whatever the patient believes is correct is an appropriate response to any question.
4. Make sure the examination room is quiet, so the patient can concentrate on your questions.
5. If family members are present, they may be helpful in "filling in" missing details.

"UNCOOPERATIVE" PATIENT

Like the "angry" or "hostile" patient, this is a difficult patient to handle. First, try to determine *why* you think the patient is being uncooperative.

Understanding the reasons for this can provide the doctor with ideas on how to gain the patient's cooperation.

Strategies for Interaction

1. Try to determine what is causing the patient to manifest uncooperative behaviors.
2. Ask patients if there is anything you can do to make them more comfortable.
3. Praise the patient for cooperative behavior.
4. Try to create a safe, secure environment for the patient.
5. Reassure patients of your interest in their well-being.

> DR. RICH: Ms. Kipp, I have been trying to get you to answer some questions that will help me understand the problem with your eyes, but you seem very hesitant to answer my questions. Is there anything that I can do to make you more comfortable? (The doctor acknowledges the patient's lack of cooperation somewhat indirectly, and asks what can be done to improve the situation for the patient.)

> MS. KIPP: You're the doctor. I don't see why *I* should have to answer questions. The reason I came to you is for you to tell me if I have a problem. So I don't see why you are asking all these questions. (The patient continues to respond in an angry tone.)

> DR. RICH: I always ask a set of questions at the start of the examination to help me determine if there are any problems. The information that you can give me will assist me in helping you. Is there anything on your mind about your eyes that you are concerned about, or anything that you would like to discuss with me? (The doctor expresses understanding, and explains the reason for the questions. The doctor tries to build a facilitative relationship by allowing the patient to voice her concerns.)

> MS. KIPP: No, I just want to know if *you* think there is anything wrong with me. Can't you just examine my eyes, and tell me what my problem is? (The patient responds angrily, and is still resistant and uncooperative.)

> DR. RICH: Ms. Kipp, you seem very resistant to my questions. Is there any reason that you are hesitant in answering my questions, or anything that I can do to make you feel more comfortable in working with me? (The doctor acknowledges the patient's resistance more directly this time.)

> MS. KIPP: Actually, I just had my eyes examined last week, and the doctor told me what *he* thought was wrong. I'm really coming to you for a second opinion, but I don't want to tell you what the other doctor found. (The patient finally expresses the cause of her resistance to the doctor. With an understanding of the patient's concern, the doctor can phrase questions in a way that does not appear to violate or threaten the patient's goals in seeking the examination.)

STRATEGIES FOR WORKING WITH "DIFFICULT" PATIENTS

Handling "difficult" patient encounters effectively is the hallmark of an expert communicator. A number of the strategies discussed in previous chapters can make these interactions more effective.

1. The doctor should remember to
   - demonstrate good listening skills,
   - display empathy,
   - make appropriate use of open-ended and closed-ended questions,
   - create a sense of safety and security in the environment,
   - understand a patient's anxiety and apprehension,
   - recognize different personality styles and ways of orienting your interactions to the individual, and
   - assure patients of your respect for their desire to be involved when management plans are determined.
2. Remember that patients are often anxious and nervous when going to the doctor. Their behaviors are frequently a reflection of the stress they experience in addressing their health care problems and concerns. Demonstrating warm, sensitive attitudes can often make patients feel more comfortable and secure.
3. Resist the temptation to become angry, hostile, or defensive in these situations. Being prepared for these situations can enable the doctor to call on constructive strategies and approaches.
4. Make appropriate use of open-ended questions, closed-ended questions, reflection, legitimation, and other communication techniques (Chapter 3). Using the appropriate strategy can facilitate interactions in these situations.
5. Reassure patients that you are listening to their concerns and are sensitive to their needs.
6. Respond to both the emotional and factual content of a patient's communications. Doctors often avoid responding to emotional cues. Ignoring affective cues can make a patient feel that the doctor is not listening, and this creates an obstacle to effective interactions.
7. Working with "difficult" patients often requires extra time and extra patience; make sure that you are generous with these resources.

QUESTIONS FOR THOUGHT

1. Give three recommendations for managing each of the following types of patients:
   a. The "silent" patient.
   b. The "rambling" patient.

    c. The "evasive" patient.

    d. The "grief" patient.

2. How would you respond to the following comments?

    a. "The last two doctors have not been able to help me. You probably won't either, but I'll let you try."

    b. "Why can't I see well with the new contact lenses you gave me last week? I waited a long time to get them, and now I'm having problems with them."

    c. "I'm in a rush to get home and I don't have time for a full examination, but I need a new reading prescription right away."

    d. "I know what's wrong with me, so you don't even have to examine me. I had a 'red' eye two years ago and the doctor gave me this prescription. (The patient takes out a tube of antibiotic ointment.) I need a new prescription for this medicine."

3. Provide three suggestions for handling each of the following types of patients:

    a. The "nervous" patient.

    b. The "malingering" patient.

    c. The "poor historian."

    d. The "uncooperative" patient.

4. Discuss the approach that the doctor can use in handling an "angry" patient.

5. Discuss reasons patients demonstrate "seductive" behaviors in the clinical environment. What would you say in response to a seductive comment or behavior? How do you handle the "seductive" patient and maintain a cordial, professional relationship?

REFERENCES

Alessandra T, O'Connor MJ. Peoplesmart. La Jolla, CA: Keynote Publishing Co., 1990.

Bramson RM. Coping with Difficult People. New York: Dell, 1981.

Cohen-Cole SA. The Medical Interview: The Three-Function Approach. St. Louis, MO: Mosby Year Book, 1991.

Groves JE. Taking care of the hateful patient. New England Journal of Medicine 298:883–887, 1978.

Keating CJ. Dealing with Difficult People. New York: Paulist Press, 1984.

Levinson D. A Guide to the Clinical Interview. Philadelphia: W.B. Saunders, 1987.

Muchnick BG, Nyman NN. The uncooperative patient: Keep cool, take charge. Review of Optometry 129(8):69–72, 1992.

ADDITIONAL READINGS

Bernstein L, Bernstein RS. Interviewing—A Guide for Health Professionals. Norwalk, CT: Appleton-Century-Crofts, 1985.

Gailmard NB. Managing the grief patient. Optometric Economics 1(8):18–22, 1991.

Leon RL. Psychiatric Interviewing: A Primer. New York: Elsevier, 1989.

Lipp MR. Respectful Treatment—A Practical Handbook of Patient Care. New York: Elsevier, 1986.

Okun BF. Effective Helping Interviewing and Counseling Techniques. Pacific Grove, CA: Brooks/Cole, 1987.

15

Communicating with Psychiatric Patients

Patients with psychiatric disorders pose a unique set of challenges to health professionals. Unless they specialize in the field, most health care workers are not trained in the management and care of patients with psychiatric disorders. The behavioral patterns and responses of these patients make it difficult to collect a case history or to conduct the clinical examination. The challenge lies in facilitating an effective interaction based on the doctor's ability to gain the cooperation and participation of the patient.

Psychiatric terms, such as "hysterical," "paranoid," or "neurotic," are often used erroneously and pejoratively by uninformed individuals. It is important for nonpsychiatric health care professionals to refrain from making psychiatric diagnoses and to be careful not to mislabel patients. Diagnosis should be left to those who are specifically trained in the complex and complicated field of psychopathology. Referral and consultation with psychologists, psychiatrists, social workers, and other mental health professionals should be initiated when a psychological or psychiatric evaluation is indicated. Effective interactions with these professionals are in the best interests of patient management (see Chapter 10).

It has been estimated that approximately 20% of medical patients suffer from significant psychiatric problems; at least half of these disorders are unidentified by physicians (Cohen-Cole 1991). It is estimated that patients with mental illness utilize twice as much nonpsychiatric medical care as patients without mental illness. There is clearly a need for nonpsychiatric professionals to be able to recognize the signs of mental illness. A number of factors can be evaluated to gain insights into a patient's mental status:

Attention span

Level of consciousness and alertness

Appearance

Speech and use of language

Mood and affect

Memory

Thought processes

The stereotypical image of the mentally ill patient as a violent, uncontrollable individual is generally untrue. In some categories, behavior can be inconsistent (e.g., borderline patients) and health care professionals should monitor a patient's behavior. By understanding the individual needs of patients with psychiatric disorders, clinicians will find that most patients can be managed effectively with a variety of patient-oriented strategies.

Six of the categories listed in the *Diagnostic and Statistical Manual of Mental Disorders* (DSM-III-R) (1987) will be discussed in this chapter: personality disorders, mood disorders (including depression), anxiety disorders and phobic neuroses, schizophrenia, somatoform disorders, and organic mental disorders (Table 15.1). Psychoactive substance abuse, another classification frequently used in psychiatry, is covered in Chapter 13 (pp. 199–201). Once the general categories of psychiatric disorders are understood, meaningful and useful strategies to facilitate good care with these individuals can be developed.

PERSONALITY DISORDERS

Personality disorders are persistent, long-term patterns of behavior that are considered socially maladaptive. These patients tend to have "alloplastic defenses"; this means that they react to stress by trying to change the external environment to support their own needs and desires (Goldman 1992). This desire to control often makes the doctor–patient encounter difficult.

Paranoid Patients

Paranoid individuals are characterized by suspicious thinking; they may believe that other people are saying or thinking bad things about them,

Table 15.1 Some categories of mental disorders

Personality disorders
    Paranoid
    Schizoid
    Schizotypal
    Antisocial
    Borderline
    Histrionic
    Narcissistic
    Avoidant
    Dependent
    Obsessive-compulsive
    Passive-aggressive

Mood disorders
    Bipolar disorders
    Depressive disorders

Anxiety disorders and phobic neuroses
    Panic disorder
    Agoraphobia
    Social phobia
    Simple phobia
    Obsessive-compulsive neurosis
    Posttraumatic stress disorder
    Generalized anxiety disorder

Somatoform disorders
    Conversion disorders (or hysterical neurosis)
    Hypochondriasis (or hypochondriacal neurosis)
    Somatization disorder

Schizophrenia
    Catatonic
    Disorganized
    Paranoid
    Undifferentiated
    Residual

Organic mental disorders
    Degenerative dementia (Alzheimer type)
    Senile dementia
      Presenile dementia
    Alcohol, drug, and substance-induced organic mental disorders
    Delirium
    Dementia
    Amnestic disorder

following them, or plotting against them. They tend to be highly attentive to any evidence that seems to corroborate their suspicions.

Paranoid individuals tend to feel easily threatened by the doctor and office staff. They may criticize the way they are being handled, or they may complain if certain services are not given to them.

Strategies for Interaction

1. Make the patient as comfortable as possible. Create a sense of safety and security (Lipkin 1987). Avoid distractions and unnecessary technical language.
2. Demonstrate respect.
3. Work with the patient's need for autonomy and self-control. Give the patient control over as many aspects of the encounter as possible (without compromising the quality of the testing). As Lipkin recommends, "You tell me," "Please make lists," and other forms of patient involvement give the patient a heightened sense of autonomy. In taking visual acuities, the doctor can show patients a large chart and give them the responsibility of choosing the smallest letters that can be seen, rather than telling them exactly which line to read.
4. Praise and support patients for the knowledge that they display.
5. When a patient's questions seem untrusting or suspicious, answer respectfully, nonjudgmentally, and factually. Becoming defensive or angry is counterproductive.
6. Use open-ended questions during the case history so patients feel comfortable expressing what they want to share; specific, focused questions may intimidate or threaten the patient.

A 37-year-old male presents for a general eye examination. His chief complaint is long-standing decreased vision in his left eye. He claims to have experienced the vision loss as the result of an incident seven years ago, in which he was arrested and hit with a police officer's club. He says that he has been to several eye doctors since then, and no one has been able to identify his problem. He adds, "I think it is part of the conspiracy against me." He talks about doctors he has visited who have been "part of the plot" against him. He also talks about people at his job who are involved in the same plan. He reports being under a psychiatrist's care, treated for "stress." He is not taking any medications, and no other medical problems are known.

DR. ROYE: Mr. Howard, I can tell that you are concerned about the vision in your left eye. I will examine you very carefully, and try to determine what is causing the problem. If you have any questions as we proceed, please feel free to ask me.

As the doctor performs the examination, the patient questions why tests are being done, and what the doctor finds. The patient is reassured that the doctor is trying to determine what is causing his symptoms.

The doctor finds that the test results do not correspond with the patient's symptom of decreased vision. The patient exhibits 20/20 visual acuity in each eye, at distance and near. Ocular health tests reveal no sign of pathology. Additional procedures, including visual field analysis, contrast sensitivity evaluation, and color vision testing reveal no decreased function in the left eye. The doctor suspects that communicating these results to the patient may be challenging and considers the approach to be used carefully.

DR. ROYE: Mr. Howard, the tests that I've done today show that both of your eyes are healthy. I'm not finding any reason for the vision in your left eye to be reduced.

MR. HOWARD: How can that be? (Pause; then he shakes his head.) You did the same tests as all the other doctors. Can't you do the right test to find the problem?

DR. ROYE: Mr. Howard, do you have any idea why you feel the vision in your left eye is decreased? (Dr. Roye recognizes that although the basis is not visual, the patient has a problem that must be recognized and addressed.)

MR. HOWARD: I think when they hit me seven years ago, something happened. I heard a noise, and I know that from then on, something changed in my eye.

DR. ROYE: What do you think can be done to restore your vision?

MR. HOWARD: Nothing. Absolutely nothing. They made sure that they got me good. I don't think anybody knows how to fix what they did.

The interaction with the patient convinces the doctor that the symptom is related to the patient's psychiatric problems. When the patient acknowledges that he has not mentioned the vision problem to his psychiatrist, Dr. Roye recommends that the patient discuss this problem. With Mr. Howard's permission, a report is sent from the optometrist to the psychiatrist.

Although the optometrist was not able to solve the patient's problem in the way the patient wanted, the optometrist was successful in forming a therapeutic relationship with the patient, and in assessing the patient's needs.

Histrionic Patients

Histrionic disorders are frequently referred to as hysterical personality styles. These patients consistently demonstrate acute emotions and strong feelings and are frequently flamboyant in language, dress, and interpersonal interactions. They may report false information or exaggerated descriptions of their symptoms stemming from their use of language or from their desire to gain added attention from the health care provider. While they may not be truly interested in intimacy, these patients may display sexual, seductive behavior to gain attention.

Strategies for Interaction

1. Demonstrate good listening and responding skills. Reassure the patient of your attention and be responsive to the patient's needs.

2. Be careful to maintain an appropriate level of concern. Excessive attention can reinforce a patient's need and expectation for additional attention.

3. Use open-ended questions to help patients feel that they have adequate opportunity to express their needs and feelings. If the patient is verbose, going to closed-ended questions may help provide some additional structure for responses.

4. Set appropriate limits in maintaining a professional relationship (see Chapter 14, pp. 213–216).

A 36-year-old female presents to the eye doctor for an examination. She is dressed in a flashy outfit. She speaks in a dramatic tone, and her thoughts are expressed in flowing detail. Her chief visual complaint involves discomfort at near.

At times during the examination, she displays flirtatious behavior in her verbal and nonverbal cues. When this happens, the doctor politely attempts to turn the conversation back to topic of the examination.

DR. WALKER: Good morning, Ms. Collins. What brings you in today?

MS. COLLINS: It's been awhile since I've seen you. You look like you've had a good summer. That's a nice tan you have.

DR. WALKER: Thank you (neutral tone). Tell me, have you had any problems with your eyes lately?

MS. COLLINS: Yes, I've noticed some changes. I could be reading my newspaper, and the letters just start to move together. I'm glad I came to see you. I know that you will be able to help me with my problem.

DR. WALKER: Tell me a little more about your problem with your vision.

MS. COLLINS: My eyes get so tired. I can be reading and the letters just start to move around. I can see the letters on the page. They are right in front of me, but they just start to dance around.

DR. WALKER: How long have you noticed this problem?

MS. COLLINS: A few months, I guess. So I decided to come to see you. It's not often that I look forward to going to the doctor, but in your case (pause)—you make me feel so good (suggestive tone).

DR. WALKER: (Returning to the topic of the examination.) Ms. Collins, do your eyes feel tired when you start to read, or does the problem occur after you're reading for awhile?

MS. COLLINS: Oh, it's fine when I start reading. But after I'm reading for awhile, that's when the letters start to move around. They just dance, dance, dance. Do you think it's something serious? Please, tell me everything. I can take it—don't spare me. I definitely want to know if something is wrong.

DR. WALKER: Well, it sounds like something we can handle, but I need to ask you some more questions and take a look at your eyes before I know for sure.

MS. COLLINS: Oh, I knew you'd be able to handle it. I thought it was something really serious. You always make me feel better when I am with you.

DR. WALKER: (The doctor realizes that the patient frequently brings the conversation back to him, and that he must return to the topic of the examination.) I'd be happy to help you with your eye problems. Are you having any trouble seeing things at distance?

MS. COLLINS: Oh no, not at all. When I'm looking at things far away, I can see forever and ever. Those glasses that you gave me are great. I think they look pretty good, too. Do you like the way they look on me?

DR. WALKER: They look fine (neutral tone). I need to ask some more questions about your vision. Do you ever see double?

MS. COLLINS: No, never double. But my eyes bother me. I was thinking the other day—I've got to get Dr. Walker to hold my hand when I'm reading. Maybe that will solve the problem!

DR. WALKER: Well, I definitely want to help you solve your vision problem, so I'm going to have to continue with the examination, and some tests to evaluate your eyes.

The doctor finds that the patient has a convergence insufficiency, which results in her problems at near. The doctor discusses a program of visual therapy that can reduce the patient's visual symptoms and allow her to use her vision more efficiently. By ignoring the suggestive behavior and maintaining a therapeutic relationship, the doctor is able to identify the patient's visual problems and determine a patient-oriented management plan.

Narcissistic Patients

It is believed that the narcissistic personality results from poor self-esteem and self-confidence. Generally unaware of their insecurity, the individual's desire for special treatment may be due to a need for respect.

Narcissistic patients are demanding patients who seek preferential treatment and special attention from the doctor and office staff. They expect their needs to be met immediately, and tend to complain if they feel that their needs are not being met.

Strategies for Interaction

1. Set an appropriate balance between reassuring the patient and setting limits. Demonstrate attention, concern, and interest in these patients

and their needs. Be aware that, in the absence of limits, the patient may take advantage of the attention.

2. Emphasize what *can* and *is* being done for the patient, rather than what *cannot* be done to accommodate their needs.

3. Give the patient some sense of control by asking what would make him or her happier (Cohen-Cole 1991).

4. Point out some of the special services provided in your office to relax and ease some of the patient's other demands.

A 49-year-old female, employed as a manager at a department store, presents to the office for a contact lens follow-up visit. She arrives at the office an hour early for her appointment expecting to be taken early. The reception room is filled with patients who have earlier appointments.

MS. JACKOBY: What a day I'm having! First they needed me in one department, and then in another. I arrived here early because I absolutely have to be out of here in a half hour. I've got another appointment this afternoon, and I'm really in a rush.

RECEPTIONIST: Ms. Jackoby, we would love to take you early if there was an available appointment, but you can see other people have been waiting. We'll try to have the doctor get to you as soon as possible. (The receptionist assures the patient that they will try to see her soon.)

MS. JACKOBY: But I'm really in a rush. Please tell the doctor I need to be taken now; I'm sure the doctor will be happy to see me.

RECEPTIONIST: Yes, the doctor is definitely looking forward to seeing you. The doctor is planning to devote adequate time to examine you carefully. (Now the receptionist is speaking of the patient's needs.)

MS. JACKOBY: Great, I really need to have my lenses checked.

RECEPTIONIST: To give you the attention you deserve, we have planned your appointment carefully. (This makes the patient feel important.) That is why we have reserved your appointment time. We would not want to cut your time with the doctor.

MS. JACKOBY: Well, of course not. But can't the doctor see me now?

RECEPTIONIST: Ms. Jackoby, the doctor is not able to see you ahead of time today. (The receptionist sets some firm limits.) But as you know, you are very important to us. It must be pretty difficult to have another appointment planned after this one. Is there anything I can do to make you more comfortable so you can wait until the doctor is ready for you? (The receptionist gives the patient some sense of control, and asks what would make her happier.)

MS. JACKOBY: Well (thinking) . . . I really would need to phone my next appointment and tell them when I will arrive.

RECEPTIONIST: Terrific. Here's the phone. Please feel free to make your call. I'm so glad that you will be able to stay, and that the doctor will be able to take care of you.

Dependent Patients

The dependent patient relies on the health care professional for emotional support and frequently presents to the doctor's office and contacts the doctor by telephone. When they receive the attention they seek, these patients often bestow abundant appreciation and praise on the doctor. This sometimes evokes favorable responses from many health professionals who find the adulation enticing. However, Cohen-Cole (1991) points out that the "brief honeymoon between the satisfied patient and doctor can fail as the patient becomes more and more dependent, and the physician tires of giving more and more time and emotional supplies."

Strategies for Interaction

1. Set firm limits and maintain a therapeutic, helping relationship.
2. Validate the patient's importance. Excessive attention, however, can be counterproductive to this continuing relationship.

> Ms. Saxon has been a patient in Dr. Mason's office for the past six months. During this time, she has frequently stopped by between appointments asking to see the doctor. She has recently started a program of vision therapy for convergence insufficiency. Her binocular problems have caused moderate discomfort and fatigue at work.
>
> Although flattered by the patient's consistent compliments and attention, the doctor realizes that the patient must become an active participant to attain optimum results from her vision therapy program and health care. Her dependent behavior must be transformed to a more responsible role. The doctor encourages Ms. Saxon to take an active role in the vision therapy program, holding the instruments herself, and reporting her own visual experiences and responses. When she notices improvements in her vision, she compliments Dr. Wright on being a good doctor. The doctor explains supportively to the patient that her success is a result of her commitment and effort, and that she should take responsibility for her work. The doctor responds in a more neutral manner to her flattering comments, encouraging her more independent actions. Over time, the dependent characteristics of the relationship decrease, and the patient demonstrates greater independence.

Obsessive-Compulsive Patients

Obsessive-compulsive patients are detail-oriented, highly structured, rigid individuals. They avoid uncertainty and ambiguity and look for organization, control, and predictability. Unlike histrionic individuals, obsessive-compulsive patients do not express emotions well, and their function revolves more around facts than feelings. Any perception of uncertainty or ambiguity may produce anxiety and insecurity.

Strategies for Interaction

1. Create a safe atmosphere. Provide the patient with detailed explanations of tests before you perform them to help the patient feel safe.
2. Clearly focused, well-defined, closed-ended questions are preferable for these patients; broad, open-ended questions may evoke confusion and anxiety.
3. Provide adequate details to satisfy the patient's need for fine detail and explanation.
4. Validate the patient's importance to you. Take the time to ask if the patient has any questions and respond to any inquiries; this can be reassuring to the patient.

> Mr. Hammel, a 39-year-old painter, presents to the doctor. The receptionist informs the doctor that the patient was upset that he was taken five minutes late for the examination.
>
> The doctor begins the case history and finds that there are no visual complaints. Now he is ready to inquire about the patient's general medical status.
>
> DR. REYES: Mr. Hammel, we have discussed your visual symptoms and your eye health. How is your general health?
>
> MR. HAMMEL: It's pretty good. No problems, for the most part.
>
> DR. REYES: Are you currently being treated by any other doctors, or followed for any conditions?
>
> MR. HAMMEL: I am seeing a doctor for some other problems. A psychologist. Dr. Jenner. (Long pause.) My wife says I get crazy when things change around me. I like the "regular" routine. Wake up at five o'clock. Go to work at seven. Lunch at noon, and home at six. There was extra traffic on the way home yesterday, and I got home twenty minutes late. I just can't take it when things don't go as planned.
>
> DR. REYES: What does Dr. Jenner say?
>
> MR. HAMMEL: Dr. Jenner is trying to help me deal with changes more easily. But it's hard.
>
> DR. REYES: I'm glad that you mentioned that to me. When we are done, I can send a report of my examination to Dr. Jenner, if you'd like.

The doctor acknowledges the patient's statement about having difficulty adjusting to change, and works to create a secure feeling for the patient with frequent explanations and reassurances. By recognizing the patient's needs, the doctor can provide optimal conditions for a productive clinical encounter. Sending a report to the patient's psychologist is in the patient's best overall interest.

Borderline Personality Disorder

Borderline personality disorder is characterized by frequent mood changes, unstable personal relationships, and impulsive behaviors. Historically, the term was used to describe a condition that "bordered" between neurosis and psychosis; it is now used to describe a personality disorder characterized by poor self-identity and ineffective personal relationships.

These patients are often hostile, angry, and demanding, and they may experience mood swings in the clinical environment. This inconsistent behavior is the most difficult aspect of dealing with these patients.

Strategies for Interaction

1. Project a positive attitude and provide support and reassurance.
2. Open-ended questions can be helpful in providing patients with a feeling that they have an adequate opportunity to express their needs and concerns.
3. Be prepared to handle the patient's sudden mood shifts. From reserved and quiet, they may become intense and hostile.
4. Set appropriate limits when patients present excessive demands.

Other Personality Disorders

Schizoid, schizotypal, antisocial, and avoidant personalities all exhibit difficulties in interpersonal relationships. In many cases, they avoid social contact. Passive-aggressive individuals characteristically demonstrate hostile behaviors in indirect, nonphysical ways.

These patients often find it difficult to trust doctors, and it may take great effort for the doctor to establish a helping relationship.

Strategies for Interaction

1. Create a safe atmosphere in the clinical environment.
2. Provide adequate time; do not rush these patients.
3. Be flexible in your approach. Try broad open-ended questions to encourage patients to express their concerns and to make them feel that they have an adequate opportunity to express their needs. Patients who do not respond well to this approach may prefer to answer simpler, closed-ended questions.
4. Provide reassurance and reinforce the patient's successful interactions in the clinical environment.

MOOD DISORDERS

Mood disorders occur when patients experience extreme shifts in moods or prolonged periods of an intense mood such as depression.

Bipolar Disorders (Manic-Depressive Disorders)

Bipolar disorders are characterized by mood shifts from extreme excitement (mania) to intense lows (depression) that can occur along a continuum of intensities from mild, to moderate and severe.

Depressive Disorders

Depressive disorders are referred to as unipolar because they consist of extended periods of depression. Sleep disturbances, changes in weight and appetite, difficulty concentrating, and feelings of worthlessness are frequent signs. Suicidal thoughts may also occur.

Major depression is characterized by patients who react to a situation or an event with (1) a disproportionate degree of sadness and despondency and (2) a failure to recover within a reasonable amount of time.

Illness and aging are frequently associated with depression. When signs of significant depression are identified, appropriate referrals to psychiatric and psychological colleagues should be made.

Strategies for Interaction

1. Respond to signs for help from these individuals by making sure that they have proper referrals to mental health care professionals.
2. Give patients adequate time to express their concerns.
3. Do not ignore a patient's affective messages. Respond to their communications along the affective dimension.
4. Demonstrate good listening skills and empathic responding.

> Mr. Lockwood is a 69-year-old retired teacher. He has enjoyed reading tremendously throughout his life, but has found that his vision has decreased extensively during the past few years. He has age-related macular degeneration in both eyes, with best corrected distance visual acuities of 20/100 in the right eye and 20/80 in the left eye. He has expressed concern and sadness over his loss. The patient has attempted to use low vision aids for reading but has been unsuccessful. At the current time, he appears unusually sad and dejected. He appears to have lost weight, and complains about not being able to sleep. On further questioning, the patient expresses intense fears about the future and his advancing age. He is visibly distressed. Although the doctor and his office

staff have been supportive of the patient, the doctor feels that this case warrants the attention of a mental health care professional.

The doctor discusses the situation with the patient and suggests a psychological evaluation. The optometrist calls a colleague to set up an appointment, offers his continued support of the patient, and invites the patient to call or return if there are any additional questions or concerns.

ANXIETY DISORDERS AND PHOBIC NEUROSES

Neurotic patients develop "autoplastic defenses" and react to stress by changing their *internal* psychological processes to avoid facing an underlying problem. Neuroses are behavior patterns that are frequently *extreme* forms of normal defense mechanisms used to handle anxiety and stress. Under pressure, the neurotic individual may rationalize that something essential, but difficult to attain, is of no significance. The patient with a neurotic disorder may have maladaptive behaviors, but he or she is still clearly in touch with reality. Anxiety disorders and phobias are frequently considered neuroses.

Panic Disorders

Panic disorders are characterized by acute anxiety attacks during which the individual may experience rapid beating of the heart, rapid breathing, perspiration, muscle tension, nausea, and intense fear. The anxiety is usually linked with specific situations, and the intensity of the anxiety is often considered out of proportion to the specific situation.

Simple and Social Phobias

Phobias are excessive fears that are intense and out of proportion to the amount of danger that is really involved. Common phobias include fear of high places (acrophobia), open places (agoraphobia), closed spaces (claustrophobia), and darkness (nyctophobia).

Strategies for Interaction

1. Create a safe atmosphere in the clinical environment.
2. Give patients adequate time to adapt to the environment and to acclimate to testing situations. Provide explanations of procedures to patients before they are done.
3. Provide reassurance to the patient, and allow patients to ask questions to alleviate concerns and worry.

PSYCHOSIS AND SCHIZOPHRENIA

Psychosis is a severe psychiatric problem. Unlike the neurotic patient who is still clearly in touch with reality, the psychotic individual demonstrates a more prominent distortion of reality. Psychotic disorders are characterized by delusions (false beliefs) and hallucinations (false perceptions that occur in the absence of appropriate stimuli).

Psychotic individuals may believe that they are someone else, often a prominent historical or religious figure (e.g., Napoleon, Adolph Hitler, Jesus Christ). They may hallucinate, hear voices, or report inappropriate visual or auditory sensations (e.g., feeling "electric rays").

Schizophrenia (a set of disorders that results in severe disturbances in thought, perception, affect, and emotion) is the most common psychotic disorder (Wilson et al. 1992). Withdrawal from social relations is common. When severe psychotic behaviors occur, the clinical examination can be difficult. Patients sometimes fade in and out of reality. It is usually feasible to examine a psychotic patient, but in rare occasions when the patient manifests psychotic behaviors it is necessary to reschedule.

Strategies for Interaction

1. Provide structure and reassurance.
2. Project a very supportive, calm manner. Avoid sudden changes, and provide explanations when changes are necessary. New procedures and strange equipment can evoke apprehension.
3. Minimize physical contact. Many psychotic patients do not like to be touched.
4. Avoid "overloading" the patient with too much information at once.
5. Plan for extra time. These encounters require patience.
6. Monitor the patient's behavior and response during the examination. Psychotic patients can become hostile at times, although this does not occur frequently.
7. Psychotic patients can usually respond to testing adequately. In certain cases, however, it may be necessary to stop and reschedule the appointment.

Mr. Woodly, a 68-year-old male, presents for an eye examination with his daughter. The patient mentions that he has been under a psychiatrist's care, diagnosed as psychotic. Although the daughter tells you that her father was resistant to coming for an eye examination initially, he is cooperative when testing begins. Ten minutes into the examination, however, he starts hearing voices. Voices and hallucinations prevent the doctor from continuing with the examination. The patient becomes angry, and his daughter calms him down. This is one of those rare cases in which the doctor has to stop and reschedule the examination to complete the remainder of testing at another time.

SOMATOFORM DISORDERS

Somatoform disorders are found in patients who report physical symptoms generally associated with disease and pathology in the absence of any organic or physiological explanation. Examples are hysterical blindness, paralysis of body parts, and internal body sensations (Wilson et al. 1992; DiMatteo 1991).

These individuals have patterns of long-standing somatic symptoms leading them to consult one doctor after another, without finding an underlying physical cause. These patients are often hospitalized and have unnecessary medical procedures and surgery. Common symptoms include shortness of breath, palpitations, dizziness, back pain, abdominal pain, and gastrointestinal problems. These patients often abuse medications as they attempt to address their symptoms.

Conversion Disorders (or Hysterical Neurosis)

In hysterical neurosis, physical symptoms appear without any underlying physical contributing factor. Symptoms may be sensory (e.g., loss of vision), motor (e.g., paralysis of a limb or a side of the body), or visceral (e.g., related to internal organs of the body such as body aches, or "lumps" in the throat). The hysterical patient must be differentiated from the malingering patient who is feigning an illness. (For more information on malingerers, see Chapter 14, pages 211–212.)

Hypochondriasis (or Hypochondriacal Neurosis)

Individuals with hypochondriacal neurosis are excessively preoccupied with their health and with various presumed disorders and conditions. They may tend to exaggerate or fabricate symptoms, so the health care professional has to be careful to look for consistency in patient reports. Symptoms and irrelevant conditions should not be suggested, and care should be taken to monitor the medications that the patient is taking. Any questions about the patient's general medical status and medical therapy should be discussed with the patient's general physician.

Strategies for Interaction

1. Provide supportive, empathic care. Patients often go from one doctor to another when they feel their symptoms are not addressed.
2. Do not suggest symptoms or pathological conditions to the patient.

3. Always inquire about what medications these patients are using. They are often taking unnecessary drugs.
4. When indicated, make sure that these patients have access to psychiatrists and other mental health care professionals.

ORGANIC MENTAL DISORDERS

Organic mental disorders are psychiatric disturbances that are associated with brain insult and can produce significant changes in behavior, memory, and attention.

A variety of neurologic and nonneurologic conditions can produce psychiatric symptoms. Drugs used in the treatment of medical conditions can also result in psychiatric problems. Organic mental disorders can be transient or permanent. Three categories of organic mental disorders will be discussed:

Delirium is characterized by a reduced attention span, disorganized thinking, perceptual disturbances, disorientation, sleep disturbances, and memory impairment. Visual hallucinations are common.

Dementia is characterized by impaired memory (short- and long-term), impaired abstract thinking and judgment, and personality changes. Other disturbances of higher cortical function (e.g., aphasia, apraxia, agnosia) may also be present.

Amnestic syndrome is characterized by impaired memory, in the absence of any other impairments in cognitive and intellectual functioning. Causes include head trauma, cerebral hemorrhage, carbon monoxide poisoning, and other incidents causing hypoxia.

Strategies for Interaction

1. Be flexible and adaptive in your approach. Take into account any impairments in perceptual function, abstract thinking, attention span, and memory.
2. If indicated, provide extra time for the patient to respond and process information.
3. Reassure the patient and foster a sense of security.
4. Inquire about the patient's medical care. Appropriate interdisciplinary communications with the patient's other health care providers can benefit the patient's overall care.

Ms. Dubart is a 79-year-old female who presents for an eye examination because she has lost her glasses. She is accompanied by a caretaker who explains that Ms. Dubart has had problems with her memory in the past year. She has had problems sleeping at night, and experiences disorientation. She is under the care of both an internist and a psychiatrist.

To interact with this patient optimally, the doctor makes a special effort to make her comfortable. The doctor also remembers the importance of forming a therapeutic relationship with both the patient and the caretaker. All case history questions are addressed to Ms. Dubart, but when she is not able to recall some information, the caretaker provides some assistance.

Aside from mild cataracts, the doctor does not identify any signs of ocular pathology. A new bifocal prescription is determined. The doctor suggests that the patient consider obtaining a spare pair of glasses, or a chain to hold the glasses around her neck. The optometrist offers to send a report to the patient's internist and psychiatrist to share useful information.

ORGANIC AND DRUG-INDUCED CAUSES OF MENTAL DISORDERS

Health professionals working with patients should be aware that various physical diseases can cause psychiatric signs and behaviors (Table 15.2).

In addition, drugs used in the treatment of medical conditions can result in psychiatric symptoms. The therapeutic drugs that most commonly produce psychiatric symptoms are Prednisone, Isoniazid, Methyldopa, NPH Insulin, Diazapam, Furosemide, Phenobarbital, Chlordiazapoxide, and Aminophylline (Lipp 1986).

When psychiatric symptoms are observed in patients with physical diseases, communicating with the patient's other doctors is valuable. When patients on drug therapies exhibit these psychiatric behaviors, it is important to communicate with the managing doctor to determine whether a modification in dose, or a change in drug choice, may be useful.

MAKING APPROPRIATE REFERRALS

For individuals who identify themselves as psychiatric patients, the best way a nonpsychiatric professional can help the patient is to

1. See that the patient is confident and comfortable in the psychiatric or psychological care that is being received.
2. Provide sources of referrals if the patient is looking for another mental health care professional.
3. Identify whether the patient is in any crisis, needing immediate attention.
4. Send a report to the psychologist providing information about the patient's condition, with any pertinent insights. (Interprofessional communications can improve clinical care.)

Table 15.2 Medical conditions that produce psychiatric symptoms

Condition	Comments
Neurological	
Alzheimer's disease	Can produce anxiety, disorientation, memory loss
Multiple sclerosis	Can produce anxiety, depression, psychosis
Parkinson's disease	Most commonly associated with depression
Myopathies	Most commonly associated with depression
Delirium	Can produce anxiety
Dementia	Can produce anxiety
Myasthenia gravis	Can produce depression
Wilson's disease	Can produce psychosis
Head trauma	Can produce anxiety, depression, psychosis
Intracranial infection (e.g., encephalitis, meningitis, neurosyphilis, HIV infection)	Can produce anxiety, depression, psychosis
Nonneurological	
Infectious diseases (e.g., infectious mononucleosis, neurosyphilis, encephalitis, meningitis)	Can produce depression, anxiety, and less commonly psychosis
Cushing's disease	Can produce depression, mania, or psychosis
Addison's disease	Can produce depression
Neoplastic disease (e.g., tumors of the lung, pancreas, brain)	Usually associated with depression, can also cause anxiety and mania
Anemia (e.g., pernicious anemia)	Can produce depression
Metabolic imbalance disorders (hypoxia, hepatic or kidney disease, diabetes mellitus)	Usually associated with anxiety, can also produce depression
Pheochromocytoma	Can produce anxiety
Vitamin deficiencies	Can produce anxiety or depression
Hyper- and hypothyroidism	Usually associated with depression; hypothyroidism can produce psychosis, often referred to as "myxedema madness"

Many patients who need psychiatric care have never attained entry into the mental health care system. By making appropriate referrals, the optometrist can help the patient gain access to important services. In addition, by learning about behaviors associated with psychiatric problems, the eye doctor can understand how to interact optimally with these patients during the vision examination.

In cases in which patients do not self-identify, nonpsychiatric professionals should not try to make a diagnosis. Identifying that a problem exists is the most important step in helping these patients. Once a referral is made to a psychological or psychiatric colleague, a diagnosis can be made. The eye doctor should not record subjective information about the patient's psychological status. Writing on the record that the patient is "hysterical" or "neurotic" can be embarrassing, and can even result in litigation if a patient sees the record at a later time. Documentation should include only objective, factual reflections of the patient's behavior or needs (see Chapter 9). Direct quotes are often helpful in this task.

STRATEGIES FOR COMMUNICATING WITH PSYCHIATRIC PATIENTS

1. Understand the categories and characteristic behaviors of psychiatric disorders. By understanding the needs of the psychiatric patient, the clinician can determine how to improve the doctor–patient interaction.
2. Show support, warmth, reassurance, and sensitivity to these patients. Many of them need to be reminded that they are in a safe environment. By making patients comfortable, the doctor can improve the patient's ability to cooperate and participate in the examination.
3. Avoid negative biases and stereotypes of patients with psychiatric problems.
4. Remember to maintain a positive attitude when dealing with these patients. Anger and other negative attitudes are counterproductive and should be avoided.
5. Unless you are trained in psychiatric diagnosis and management, refrain from making psychiatric diagnoses and evaluations.
6. Effective interdisciplinary communications can result in optimal care for these patients; refer when indicated.

QUESTIONS FOR THOUGHT

1. Explain the differences between the "neurotic" and "psychotic" patient. Under what circumstances would the clinical examination be difficult with each of these patients?
2. Discuss three strategies for handling (a) a paranoid patient, (b) an obsessive-compulsive patient.
3. Discuss two strategies for handling (a) a histrionic patient, (b) a narcissistic patient.

4. Why do many health care professionals find "dependent" patients appealing? What are the risks of encouraging "dependent" behavior in a patient? What are the best recommendations for handling this type of patient?
5. You examine a patient who appears to be highly anxious, speaks with great intensity when describing work, and appears stressed on other topics. Would you discuss this with the patient, or just deliver the eye care services sought? If the patient seemed inordinately anxious, and you felt that additional attention was required, how would you handle this situation?
6. You examine a patient and determine that the diagnosis is hysterical blindness. You suggest that an appointment be made to see a psychologist or psychiatrist. The patient assures you that the problem is not psychological, and is very resistant to your recommendation. You are confident of your diagnosis. How do you motivate this patient to follow your recommendation of seeing a psychologist or psychiatrist?
7. What are organic mental disorders? How can the doctor provide optimal care for the patient with these problems?
8. List four cues that reveal a patient's mental health status and can be easily observed by the nonpsychiatric health care professional.

REFERENCES

American Psychiatric Association: Diagnostic and Statistical Manual of Mental Disorders (DSM-III-R), 3rd ed. (revised). American Psychiatric Association, 1987.

Cohen-Cole SA. The Medical Interview: The Three-Function Approach. St. Louis, MO: Mosby Year Book, 1991.

DiMatteo MR. The Psychology of Health, Illness, and Medical Care. Pacific Grove, CA: Brooks/Cole, 1991.

Goldman HH. Review of General Psychiatry. Norwalk, CT: Appleton & Lange, 1992.

Lipkin M. The Medical Interview and Related Skills. In Branch WT, ed., Office Practice of Medicine. Philadelphia: W.B. Saunders, 1987.

Lipp MR. Respectful Treatment: A Practical Handbook of Patient Care. New York: Elsevier Science Publishing, 1986.

Wilson GT, O'Leary KD, Nathan P. Abnormal Psychology. Englewood Cliffs, NJ: Prentice-Hall, 1992.

ADDITIONAL READINGS

Davis K, Klar H, Coyle JT. Foundations of Psychiatry. Philadelphia: W.B. Saunders, 1991.

Dubin WR, Weiss KJ, Zeccardi JA. Organic brain syndrome: The psychiatric imposter. Journal of the American Medical Association 249:60–65, 1983.

Leon RL. Psychiatric Interviewing: A Primer. New York: Elsevier, 1989.

Othmer E, Othmer S. The Clinical Interview Using DSM-III-R. Washington, DC: American Psychiatric Association Press, 1989.

Robins LN, Regier DA (eds.). Psychiatric Disorders in America: The Epidemiologic Catchment Area Study. New York: Macmillan, 1991.

Shea SC. Psychiatric Interviewing: The Art of Understanding. Philadelphia: W.B. Saunders, 1988.

Stoudemire A (ed.). Clinical Psychiatry for Medical Students. Philadelphia: Lippincott, 1990.

16

Communicating with Pediatric Patients

Examining children can be very challenging, and very rewarding. Some clinicians are so uncomfortable at the thought of working with children that they avoid seeing any pediatric patients in their practices. Some are so enthralled with the doctor–pediatric patient interaction that they specialize in infants' and children's vision. All clinicians who have had experience in working with children are aware that communicating well with these patients can make the pediatric encounter a much more pleasant and productive experience.

Good communication skills can help build doctor–patient rapport with young patients. This is especially important since many children feel threatened when they go to a doctor's office. Gaining a child's trust can go a long way toward gaining the child's cooperation for the examination.

One of the greatest challenges in working with children is recognizing, and understanding, the different needs that they have at different ages. Erikson (1963) and Piaget (1954) described the different behaviors and needs of children at different stages. These behavioral variations can be observed in pediatric patients. To be effective, the clinician's interaction with a two-year-old is very different from the interaction with a nine-year-old, which, in turn, is very different from the interaction with a 13-year-old. The models and stages of child development can provide the doctor with insights into how to work with children at each of these age levels. In this chapter, an examination of the models and specific applications to the clinical environment will be made.

Contrary to the old myth that children cannot have eye examinations until they are able to read, there are many optometric techniques that have been recognized as valuable in the pediatric eye examination; however, the equipment and procedures alone are not adequate to ensure a successful clinical encounter. Proficiency in the aspects of good communication, in combination with competence in the procedures and techniques used in the examination of infants and children, can provide the clinician with the optimal skills to deal with young patients effectively.

Questions for the pediatric case history are presented in Appendix B.6. In addition to the typical set of questions asked in an optometric case history (see Chapter 2), the pediatric case history includes specific questions about school performance, birth history, and developmental milestones. These questions can help identify visual and perceptual problems that are important to detect early. Developmental milestones and approximate ages are presented in Table 16.1.

WORKING WITH PEDIATRIC PATIENTS

Understanding the sequence of development from birth through adolescence and early adulthood can assist the clinician in developing effective strategies for working with pediatric patients. Stages of development (Table 16.2) can help the doctor understand a child's behavior and activity at various ages. Familiarity with these stages can also help the doctor understand how to interact and develop rapport with children. Six categories of pediatric patients are discussed, with recommendations that can assist the doctor with patients in each category. (Categories similar to those developed by Erikson are discussed below; since behavior at eye examinations tends to change dramatically at around the age of 8 to 9 months, the age guidelines for the first two categories are adjusted to assist the eye care practitioner in predicting and understanding these behaviors.)

Infant—Birth to 9 Months

Even from birth, infants are sensitive to nonverbal cues and paralanguage. Touch can be a particularly effective way of communicating with an infant and conveying a sense of security to the child. Trust is extremely important for infants, who may start to cry if they sense any change or disparity from what is normal, or routine, to them. Being in a new environment—the doctor's office—can be a challenge, and being around new people—the doctor and office staff—can also be overly taxing, if too much stimulation is provided at once.

Table 16.1 Developmental milestones

Approximate Age[a]	Developmental Milestones
2 months	Laughs, smiles spontaneously
3 months	Rolls over
$3\frac{1}{2}$ months	Reaches for object
4 months	Makes cooing and gurgling sounds
$5\frac{1}{2}$ months	Sits without support Turns in response to voice
6 months	Stands holding on Plays peek-a-boo Shows good visual tracking and convergence
6–9 months	Babbles, imitates common sounds
8–9 months	Starts to show "stranger anxiety" in the presence of unfamiliar individuals; shows distress when separated from mother (or mother figure) until about 20 months
8–10 months	Creeps and crawls
9–10 months	Pulls self to stand
$9\frac{1}{2}$–10 months	Walks holding on to furniture
10 months	Stands momentarily, without holding on Says dada or mama
$11\frac{1}{2}$ months	Stands alone well
12 months	Walks
13 months	Says a few words (other than dada or mama)
17 months	Walks stairs
20 months	Combines words into two-word phrases
2 years	Uses three-word sentences Starts to show preference for handedness, which is usually well established by $4\frac{1}{2}$ to 5 years
$2\frac{3}{4}$ years	Says first and last name
7 years	Knows left/right on self
9 years	Knows left/right on others

[a]Some age estimates from Frankenberg WK, Dodds JB. Denver Developmental Screening Test. University of Colorado Medical Center, 1969.

Clinical recommendations: To build doctor–patient rapport, use touch and paralanguage.. Even if infants do not understand everything you say, they can sense *how* you speak to them and *how* you interact with them. Preferential looking is usually a valuable technique at this age, although it may become more difficult at about 8 to 9 months, when the child becomes more interested in the environment. Brightly colored targets and auditory

Table 16.2 Stages of personality development[a]

Stage	Age (in years)	Description
Trust vs. mistrust	Birth–1	Infant needs a sense of security and trust; new conditions can create uncertainty and mistrust
Autonomy vs. shame	1–3	Child is striving for a sense of autonomy and is working to master physical environment; when child reaches beyond limits of independence, anxiety can occur
Initiative vs. guilt	3–5	Child has developed a sense of autonomy and begins to join in and initiate activities with other children; efforts to interact with others and environment may result in frustration
Industry vs. inferiority	5–11	Child strives to meet demands of school and home, and works to achieve accomplishment
Identity vs. role confusion	11–18	Child is developing a sense of identity, and integrating various roles (child, sibling, student) into a self-image
Intimacy vs. isolation	18–40	Individual learns to build and maintain commitment and intimacy in relationship with another person
Generativity vs. stagnation	40–65	Individual seeks satisfaction in family, career, community activities
Integrity vs. despair	65+	Individual reviews life accomplishments; finds one's meaning in life, and accepts mortality

[a]Erikson EH. Childhood and Society. New York: Norton, 1963.

reinforcement on visual targets (e.g., bells on a toy used as a fixation target for motilities or cover test) can be helpful in attracting and maintaining a child's attention. Work quickly to prevent the child from fatiguing. Do not be afraid to have the child return if all of the information cannot be gathered at one visit. Avoid scheduling examinations during the child's regular nap time, or feeding time, since the child may be less cooperative during these times (see Case 16.1).

Toddler—9 Months to 3 Years

At this stage, the child may become more interested in the physical environment, and easily distracted from a specific target or task. The child may ignore dull, stationary targets, and examine the environment around him or her. The child at this stage may experience "stranger fear" and "separation anxiety." The child has usually formed a social attachment to one person, or a small group of selected individuals (e.g., parents, caretakers); separation from these individuals may result in distress for these children, who frequently cry and fret in their absence. Toddlers may feel vulnerable and threatened in a new territory.

Clinical recommendations: Be sensitive to the child's need for reassurance. To avoid "separation anxiety," it may be very helpful to have the accompanying parent or caretaker stay within the child's view during the clinical examination, or to have the child sit on the caretaker's lap. It is often helpful to tell young patients what you are going to do, before you start doing it, so they know what to expect. ("I'm going to shine a light in your eye now to make sure your eyes are very healthy.") Work quickly and efficiently to keep the child from fatiguing. Do not be afraid to have the child return if all of the information cannot be gathered at one visit. Continue to avoid scheduling the clinical examination during the child's normal nap time or feeding time (see Case 16.2).

Preschooler—3 to 5 Years

The child at this stage shows greater independence and greater development and understanding of language. This child shows greater initiative, and may like to explore the environment. Socialization also develops, and the child becomes more interested in other children and adults in his or her environment.

Clinical recommendations: Because of the development of language skills, and the improved understanding of language, the child at this age may be asked to be more involved in the case history. Even if the information that the child gives is not helpful, involving the child can help to build doctor–patient rapport. Children at this age are often very curious and may want to touch or look at a piece of equipment before it is used on them. Letting a child hold, or look at, instruments and pieces of equipment can be very reassuring and pleasing to a child. Give the child adequate time to respond to the doctor's questions and tests during the examination, but work efficiently to prevent fatiguing. Do not be afraid to have the child return if all of the information cannot be gathered at one visit (see Case 16.3).

School-Age Child—5 to 11 Years

The child at this stage shows even greater independence, and has an improved ability to express thoughts and use language. Problems in school may be reflective of vision problems, learning problems, and/or perceptual, developmental problems, so the case history should explore the child's function and level of achievement in school.

Clinical recommendations: This child can usually provide useful information in the case history, and may be able to discuss some visual symptoms and difficulties. The parent or caretaker may provide additional information. The doctor may benefit by listening and addressing questions to both the child and the accompanying adult (see Case 16.4).

Adolescent—11 to 18 Years

Adolescents usually want to be treated like adults, and the doctor can build doctor–patient rapport effectively by treating these patients respectfully and maturely.

Clinical recommendations: This patient can usually respond to most of the case history questions. The accompanying adult can sometimes provide additional information, especially with regard to family ocular and medical history, but it is important for the doctor not to make the adolescent feel unimportant or childish by inquiring about further information from the parent. Patients at this age can usually respond to the typical adult testing sequence (see Case 16.5).

Young Adult—18 to 21 Years

These patients typically respond to the full adult testing sequence without a problem, and can generally provide responses to the full case history. Accompanying adults can sometimes provide additional family history, and school/developmental history, but the young adult is usually fairly competent in providing responses for most of the other case history questions.

Clinical recommendations: The doctor can build doctor–patient rapport, and learn more about the patient's needs, by showing an interest in this patient's preferred activities. Young adults will frequently mention their academic plans, and thoughts about their occupational goals. Well-established doctor–patient rapport at this age can solidify the young adult's interest in ongoing clinical care, and can encourage the patient to continue to return regularly for routine eye care in subsequent adult years (see Case 16.6).

LEARNING ABOUT THE PATIENT

As the doctor gets to know the patient, special attention should be paid to finding out about the patient's cognitive, physical, perceptual, and social development. All of these may impact on how the child uses her eyes, and how the doctor will test her.

It is important to continue to develop rapport during the examination. Sometimes the doctor can facilitate the child's continued participation and cooperation by encouraging the child. Children often want reassurance that they are doing the right thing, and providing this reassurance can be a valuable component in building doctor–patient rapport. "You're doing just fine, keep going" or "You're doing great. Now read the letters on the bottom line" are "encouragers" that can help motivate the child to continue to cooperate. Positive feedback is helpful in building rapport, and in maintaining a child's cooperation throughout a full examination.

Some clinicians and office staff avoid talking to very young children and infants, assuming that their level of verbal comprehension is very limited. This can be counterproductive, since infants can understand nonverbal cues and affective cues although they may not extract full meaning from a verbal message.

In addition, the doctor should be conscious of building rapport with both the child and the caretaker. Both individuals are important in the outcome of this patient encounter. Although eye contact is often stressed with parents and caretakers, developing a caring relationship with both persons is important in building success. The effective clinician is conscious of maintaining a proper balance of communication between the caretaker and child.

Observing how the parent (or caretaker) and child interact can often provide the doctor with cues about how to interact successfully with the child. Observing the parent–child interaction can also provide the clinician with some insights on the potential for compliance for this child and family. If there is a sense of cooperation between parent and child, and between the doctor and each individual, the odds for compliance may be greater. If a doctor makes recommendations, and feels that support from the parent or caretaker is not present, then the doctor may want to take additional time to explain and discuss the recommendations to increase compliance.

The clinician should also be aware of a child's emotional responses to the doctor's recommendations. A child's cooperation in wearing glasses or in wearing a patch for amblyopia therapy may depend on the child's response to those interventions. The child's response to wearing glasses may be affected by friends, classmates, and other family members, as well as by the fact that "four-eyes" and other negative terms for children who wear glasses are still around (Terry 1992). Factors that influence an individual's health beliefs and behaviors have been discussed previously (Chapters 7 and 12). The reactions of parents, family, and classmates should be considered when interventions involving glasses, patching routines, and surgery are initiated. A particularly challenging situation occurs when a child is seriously disabled or visually impaired. Parents who are coping with these types of diagnoses may experience many of the emotions of the grief process including shock, denial, anger, bargaining, depression, and guilt. Clinicians can be instrumental in helping parents learn to accept and manage productively with these situations.

Working with children demonstrates that communication with a patient who does not fully understand the verbal content of the message does not mean that communication is not possible. Implementing appropriate strategies at the proper age levels can help the doctor interact successfully and productively with the pediatric patient.

Case 16.1

Johnny is $7\frac{1}{2}$ months old and is brought to the optometrist's office by his parents. His mother expresses concern that she has noticed Johnny's right eye turn in since birth. According to his mother, he responds well to visual targets, and does not appear to have difficulty seeing. The chief concern for her visit is the eye turn. This is Johnny's first eye examination.

Dr. Becker greets Johnny and his mother in the reception room in a warm, friendly tone. She makes sure to make eye contact with Johnny, and when Johnny smiles in response to her warm greeting, she touches Johnny's shoulder. (The doctor uses eye contact, touch, and paralanguage to build rapport. Before starting any examination procedures or picking up any instruments the doctor establishes a warm, secure interaction with the child.)

A full pediatric case history is gathered. The doctor works quickly to try to get as much done before the child fatigues, making sure to maintain a friendly interaction with Johnny throughout the examination. The child sits on his mother's lap during externals and other procedures to allow him to keep close contact with her. For the cover test and externals, the doctor uses brightly colored targets to maintain Johnny's attention. She switches targets at times to keep the child's interest. By proceeding rapidly and efficiently from one test to the next, Dr. Becker is able to obtain all of the necessary information. (In cases in which the child fatigues or starts to cry, it may be advisable to have the patient return at another date to continue testing.)

Case 16.2

Mary is a $2\frac{1}{2}$-year-old child. Her parents bring her for her first routine eye examination. They recall that she had frequent discharges from her left eye until she was about 8 months old, but these have ceased. There are no current ocular symptoms or complaints.

A child of Mary's age is more responsive to the clinical environment than children in the younger age category. Dr. Becker takes a special effort to make young children feel welcome and secure in the office by having a children's corner with toys in the reception room. She greets the child in the reception room and, as in the previous case, makes sure to establish a rapport with the child and parent before any testing is started. Again, brightly colored targets help to maintain the child's attention. Verbal feedback (e.g., "You're doing great"; "You're doing just fine") with supportive paralanguage can help to reassure the child and encourage participation. The child can either sit on the parent's lap, or in the chair, depending on the doctor's judgment and the child's preference. If the doctor notices the child becoming anxious, responding quickly to provide assurance can enable the exam to continue. Keeping the parent close by can reduce the likelihood of "separation anxiety."

Case 16.3

Ben is a $4\frac{1}{2}$-year-old child. His parents brought him in because he is going to be starting school. Both of his older brothers wear glasses full-time, and the parents want to be sure Ben is visually prepared to enter school. They report that he sits close to the television, but no other visual problems are observed.

Dr. Becker is aware that a child this age likes to show increased independence. She directs many of the case history questions to Ben, letting the parents fill in any additional details. Ben sits in the examination chair alone. Before starting any clinical procedures, the doctor tells him:

> I'm going to do a number of tests to check how well you see, Ben. I'm going to tell you about each test before I do it. If you have any questions, you can stop and ask me.

The doctor sets up a safe environment for the child, and gives him a sense of some control by letting him know that he can ask questions if he has any concerns. Dr. Becker tries to explain procedures before she does them. When getting ready to perform ophthalmoscopy, she says the following:

> Ben, I'm going to shine a light in the back of your eyes to make sure they're nice and healthy. This is what the light looks like. (She shines the circle of light in the palm of his hand, so Ben can see that the light is safe.)

When she senses any apprehension she slows down, answers questions, and provides reassurance to make sure the child remains comfortable.

Case 16.4

Martha is an 8-year-old child in the third grade. Her parents brought her for an eye examination because she is doing poorly in school. She is below grade level in reading and mathematics. They report that she still reverses letters, and makes errors in copying from the blackboard to her notebook.

Dr. Becker addresses case history questions to Martha, and lets the parents fill in additional details as appropriate. The doctor makes an effort to treat a child of this age level as maturely and respectfully as possible. She provides positive reinforcement and encouragement when the child participates. Supportive paralanguage, touch, and eye contact make the child feel comfortable and secure, without making her feel that she is being treated as a child. In addition to the general pediatric examination, Dr. Becker does a perceptual-developmental work-up. As with all school-age children, she asks the parents' permission to send copies of a report to the child's pediatrician, teacher, and school nurse.

Case 16.5

Mark is a 12-year-old male in the seventh grade. He comes in for an examination because his parents say that he has always had difficulty with colors. When he was younger, he had trouble identifying colors. Now, they notice that he has trouble picking out clothes that match. His father and uncle have a history of color blindness, but his two older brothers have no problem. The doctor directs all of the case history questions to Mark, and he is able to respond to most of the questions himself; when he is uncertain and glances over at his parents for assistance on some medical history questions, the doctor then looks to them, too, for their response. In the adolescent age range, some doctors like to have the parents sit in on the examination, and some prefer not to. The decision is best left to the doctor's judgment, and the parents' and child's preferences.

Case 16.6

Robert is an 18-year-old student. He is having trouble seeing the blackboard with his current glasses, and thinks that he may need a new prescription. Very little has to be done to orient this examination from the adult sequence. The greatest service the doctor can do for this patient is to inquire about the patient's visual needs at this age, such as schoolwork, sports, and driving. In addition, the doctor can reinforce this patient's understanding of the importance of routine eye care in the future.

STRATEGIES FOR INTERACTION

1. Establish and develop doctor–patient rapport at an age-appropriate level. In discussing pediatric examinations, it has been said that "the most important part of the examination is the time spent establishing a rapport with the child" (Hebeler 1987). The impact of the doctor–

patient rapport cannot be minimized. It is also important to build rapport with the accompanying parent or caretaker.

2. Involve the child in the case history as much as possible.

3. Maintain eye contact with the child, and use touch and paralanguage, as appropriate, to interact with the patient.

4. Consider how communication affects the outcome of clinical tests and procedures. Select age-appropriate testing techniques for infants and children (preferential looking, tumbling E charts, picture charts).

5. Consider not wearing a white coat when examining pediatric patients. Children often associate white coats with injections and other uncomfortable clinical experiences.

6. The clinical encounter starts as soon as the patient walks into the doctor's office. Have toys and books in the reception room to make a child comfortable as soon as the child arrives at the office.

7. A vulnerable time for the child occurs when he or she is called from the reception room to be taken into the examination room. (The child may have become comfortable in the reception room, but the fear of the unknown about the yet unseen examination room exists.) Many doctors like to come out to the examination room themselves to greet the child and the accompanying caretaker, rather than having someone else bring the child into the examination room. By greeting the patient in the reception room, and establishing rapport with the child, the doctor helps to build a sense of trust and security for the child.

8. Work quickly and efficiently. Be flexible in selecting tests and in changing the order of the examination sequence to meet the needs of the patient. Do not be afraid to have the child return to complete the examination if necessary.

9. To develop a deeper understanding of the child, be conscious of the child's cognitive, physical, perceptual, and social development.

10. Be observant of the parent–child interaction and of other cues to family dynamics. This can provide the doctor with insights into how to communicate optimally with the patient and the patient's family.

11. Be alert to signs of child abuse when examining children and take appropriate steps if indications are observed (see Chapter 13, pp. 190–194).

12. In addition to building rapport with the child, it is imperative to build rapport with the parent or caretaker. It is also important to maintain an appropriate balance of communication with both the child and the accompanying adult.

13. Do *not* schedule clinical examinations for infants and children during their normal nap time or feeding time, since this can interfere with a child's cooperation and responsiveness.

QUESTIONS FOR THOUGHT

1. Infants from birth to nine months have limited communication abilities compared to older children. Discuss effective ways of communicating with infants in this age group.
2. A parent brings a $3\frac{1}{2}$-year-old child in for an examination. The child is crying, and very frightened, in the reception room. What can you do to facilitate the examination of this child?
3. Children are often afraid of going to the doctor's office. What steps can you take in your clinical environment to make the visit more pleasant and reassuring for children who come to your practice?
4. In your clinical examination, you identify that an $8\frac{1}{2}$-year-old child has an accommodative infacility and a divergence insufficiency. You also find that the child has perceptual-developmental lags. This is consistent with the report of the child's poor school performance in reading and mathematics. How can you best motivate this child to cooperate with vision therapy and perceptual training?
5. You examine a $5\frac{1}{2}$-year-old child and find that the child is a refractive amblyope. You recommend glasses and a patching routine. Because of fear of teasing from friends the child does not want to wear glasses and is very resistant to the suggestion of patching. It is clear to you that compliance is questionable. You understand the importance of your intervention for this amblyopic patient. How can you motivate this patient?
6. Discuss methods of developing doctor–patient rapport with children in the following age ranges:
    a. birth to nine months
    b. nine months to three years
    c. three to five years
    d. five to 11 years
    e. 11 to 18 years.
7. How can you teach children about the importance of routine eye care? How can you help them develop good visual habits, and learn about the value of lifelong vision care?

REFERENCES

Erikson EH. Childhood and Society. New York: Norton, 1963.

Hebeler J. The pediatric patient. In Guckian JC, ed., The Clinical Interview and Physical Examination. Philadelphia: Lippincott, 1987.

Piaget J. The Construction of Reality in the Child. New York: Basic Books, 1954.

Terry RL. A study of children's reactions to eyeglasses. Contact Lens Spectrum 7(4):25–27, 1992.

ADDITIONAL READINGS

Enzer NB. Interviewing children and parents. In Enelow AJ, Swisher SN, eds., Interviewing and Patient Care. New York: Oxford University Press, 1986.

Press LJ, Moore ED. Clinical Pediatric Optometry. Boston: Butterworth-Heinemann, 1993.

Rosenbloom AA, Morgan MW. Principles and Practice of Pediatric Optometry. Philadelphia: Lippincott, 1990.

Rouse MW, London R. Development and perception. In Barresi B, ed., Ocular Assessment. Boston: Butterworth-Heinemann, 1984: 165–185.

17

Communicating with Patients from Special Populations

Patients from special populations have been underserved by the health care community for many years. In the past, many health care providers have been hesitant to work with patients with special needs and provide extensive reasons for not doing so. In many cases, the apprehension has been related to the potentially difficult interaction with the patient: "I wouldn't know how to test the patient," "I wouldn't be able to get clinical data," and, most commonly, "What if the patient is not able to speak?"

While communication with special needs patients may be difficult, it is not unachievable. The options and technology available to enhance the communications abilities of patients from special populations have expanded tremendously in recent years. Interdisciplinary communication is an essential component of the optimal care of patients from special populations (Chapter 10). Communication with family members, caretakers, and other professionals can increase the doctor's understanding of the patient's situation and needs.

To be effective, the clinical examination of the patient with special needs has to be oriented to the abilities of the individual patient (Ettinger 1991). Each patient has a unique profile of personal characteristics that will determine how the patient functions in the world and, specifically, how the patient responds to clinical testing procedures and interventions.

By learning to identify a patient's skills and abilities and to understand and utilize the methods of communicating with special patients, the doctor can be more effective in examining and providing services.

Disabilities can be congenital or acquired, stable or progressive. They can involve physical, cognitive, psychological, emotional, sensory, perceptual, and behavioral problems. Disabilities are often accompanied with a new set of terms and words. Knowing the terminology used with specific classifications is useful in working with patients. Doctors who work with patients with cerebral palsy can benefit by understanding the meaning of terms such as hemiplegia, paraplegia, and quadriplegia. Health care professionals who work with patients who have had brain damage can develop a greater understanding of their patients' abilities by understanding the terms aphasia, apraxia, and agnosia.

Most categories of disabilities can be described by a primary problem, and associated problems that sometimes occur. In cerebral palsy, the primary problem is a motor problem; associated problems that may accompany the primary one include mental retardation, sensory problems (e.g., vision, hearing), perceptual problems, and behavioral problems. It is the combination of factors that determines the patient's overall function.

In categories in which the primary disability is not visual, the importance of good visual care must not be minimized. A key strategy in working with patients from special populations is to "maximize their abilities" rather than concentrate on their limitations. If a patient already disabled by a hearing impairment develops a visual problem that is ignored and remains untreated, a secondary, unnecessary disability is imposed on the patient. Good vision care for patients with disabilities allows patients to make optimal use of their vision and visual abilities.

Patients with special needs have been underserved in the past. There is so much that eye care professionals can do to help them. It is in this spirit that this chapter is written.

DISABILITY VERSUS HANDICAP

In Chapter 13, definitions of visual impairments, visual disabilities, and visual handicaps were discussed. The general terms of impairment, disability, and handicap are frequently used with patients from special populations. To summarize:

An *impairment* is a limitation of a basic function (e.g., decreased visual or auditory acuity).

A *disability* is a decrease in the ability to perform various tasks, as a result of an impairment (e.g., inability to drive, write, watch television).

A *handicap* is the limitation that people feel their disability imposes on them; it is a perceived disadvantage that occurs in response to a disability.

It is possible for a person to be disabled, but not handicapped. Ayrault (1977) points out that a disability becomes a handicap only when it limits an individual from fulfilling a task, from doing what he or she wants to do, or becoming what he or she wants to become.

The way an individual views the disability is influenced, to some extent, by those around him. Holzhauser (1986) comments that those who are affected by the disability may add certain components to the definition of disability. A teacher may add that a disability "poses extra challenges as the student tries to learn." A parent may add that it "puts a strain on family living."

In addition, Holzhauser points out that how individuals view their own disability will affect how others view them. If, when they think about themselves, the first thing that comes to mind is their disability, there is a good chance that others will identify them strongly by their disability, too. Self-image and self-esteem affect how people interact with others. Holzhauser points out that on meeting someone, she would not want to say "Hi, I'm Gillian Holzhauser. I'm legally blind." A disability is a characteristic of the person, but it does not identify the individual, *unless the patient perceives it that way.*

Many people focus on what the individual *cannot* do. Individuals with multiple disabilities are often called multiply handicapped; this term emphasizes the effect of the disability. (Why are they not called, as an alternative, multiply *abled* for what they can do?) Helpful management strategies for the health care professional focus on what the patient *can* do, and they build on the strengths of the individual.

Attitudes of patients, family, friends, and health care providers have a significant impact on how patients manage with disabilities.

FAMILIES' RESPONSES TO DISABILITIES

Aside from the family members' participation during the clinical encounter, it is important to consider their responses to the disability. Parents who have recently been informed of a child's disability often go through emotional responses such as shock, denial, anger, and guilt. At first, they may focus more on what the child *cannot* do; they may mourn the loss of the "perfectly intact" child that they had expected and planned. Many parents become readily adaptable to their situation, and focus on what can be done.

Responses of siblings must be considered as well. Siblings may be jealous of the extra attention demanded by a brother's or sister's disabling condition. Some patients with disabilities may use the powerful "sick role" to maintain control over family activities and interactions (Shindell 1988).

In developing intervention plans and strategies, it is important to consider the response of family members to the situation.

BUILDING RAPPORT WITH PATIENTS, FAMILY, AND CARETAKERS

When working with patients with disabilities, it is important to communicate with family members, as well as patients with the disability. When disabled patients present to the doctor's office with family members and caretakers, health care professionals often speak to the family member more than they do to the patient. This is particularly true in the case of nonverbal patients.

As described in earlier chapters in which communication involves multiple individuals (Chapters 1, 13, 16), the doctor must develop a therapeutic rapport with both the parents (or caretaker) *and* the patient. When patients with disabilities are ignored in deference to their relatives, they are treated as "nonpersons." Adults with disabilities are often treated as children. The health care professional must build therapeutic relationships with both the patient and family members or caretakers to avoid this common problem in communications.

In addition to gathering optimum information, it is essential to remember that family members and caretakers often have significant influence on compliance. They are often the ones who have to arrange to take the patient for follow-up testing, or vision therapy sessions. If the family member does not have confidence in the doctor, compliance may be compromised.

Bailey et al. (1986) and Linder (1990) discussed the idea of "family-focused" programs as opposed to "child-focused" plans. "Family-focused" programs consider the needs of the family in relation to the disabled child. Focusing *only* on the individual with the disability may lead the doctor to formulate plans that are inappropriate for a family relationship. By involving family members and caretakers, health care professionals can design clinical management plans that are more suitable and realistic to a patient's life style and family situation.

ATTITUDES OF DOCTORS TOWARD PATIENTS WITH DISABILITIES

Doctors must also consider their own responses to parents and individuals with disabilities. Seligman and Seligman (1980) identified five negative attitudes of health care providers that can result in adversarial relationships with parents of disabled children:

1. Feeling sympathy, pity, fear, or hostility toward the child or the parents;
2. Demonstrating a feeling of hopelessness or hostility toward the situation;

3. Overidentification with the patient's or parent's position, reinforcing denial of the situation;
4. Viewing parental or patient observations as untrustworthy or meaningless;
5. Viewing parents or patients as emotionally disturbed.

Clearly, all of these responses are counterproductive to the situation. Health care providers need to convey respect and concern to parents and patients to obtain their trust.

As described in earlier chapters in which communication involves multiple individuals, the doctor must develop a therapeutic rapport with both the parents *and* the child. Accompanying caretakers must receive adequate attention and positive regard.

PRIMARY AND ASSOCIATED PROBLEMS

All categories of disabilities have primary characteristics. In cerebral palsy, the primary problem is a motor problem. Associated problems include mental retardation, perceptual deficits, sensory problems, and behavioral disturbances (Ettinger 1991). To understand how to interact with the patient, it is essential to understand the patient's primary and associated problems. It is common to focus on the main problem. Ignoring associated problems can make the health care professional less effective in interacting with the patient.

Associated Visual Problems

Optometrists have learned a lot more about the vision problems of patients from special populations in recent years. They have worked with patients with cerebral palsy, mental retardation, Down syndrome, autism, and other classifications. In each of these categories, patterns of ocular problems have been identified. In many cases, the prevalence of visual problems is high. Understanding the associated ocular anomalies of these classifications can prepare the eye doctor to examine these patients, and to be alert to specific types of problems that may exist (Table 17.1).

Cerebral Palsy

It is estimated that there are approximately 500,000 individuals with cerebral palsy in the United States. Patients with cerebral palsy have a high prevalence of strabismus, amblyopia, significant refractive errors, oculomotor dysfunction, accommodative deficits, and visual perceptual problems

TABLE 17.1 Descriptions of special population classifications

Category	Description/Cause	Associated Ocular Anomalies
Cerebral palsy[a]	A motor problem caused by damage to the motor centers of the brain (prenatal, perinatal, or postnatal). Can be caused by genetic, metabolic, infectious, toxic, or traumatic conditions	Strabismus Amblyopia High refractive errors Accommodative deficits Oculomotor dysfunction Visual–perceptual deficits
Hearing impaired[b]	Loss of hearing can be congenital or acquired, and can result from vascular, metabolic, infectious, degenerative, and toxic conditions. (The accompanying list describes ocular changes in congenitally hearing-impaired individual.)	Strabismus High refractive errors Usher's syndrome (retinitis pigmentosa associated with hearing loss)
Autism[c]	A behavioral syndrome characterized by four criteria: delayed or atypical development, atypical responses to sensory stimuli (including hyper- and hyporeactivity), disturbances of speech and communications (including nonverbal communications and echolalia in verbal children), and marked impairments in social and interpersonal interactions. Autism occurs four times more often in males than females. The exact cause is uncertain; however, neurobiological and central nervous system dysfunctions have been suggested	Typical visual behaviors include staring at lights ("light gazing") and objects, gaze avoidance, limited or absent eye contact Strabismus Refractive errors Impaired pursuit and OKN responses
Mental retardation[d]	Significantly subaverage intellectual functioning. Can be caused by genetic, metabolic, infectious, toxic, or traumatic conditions. Often associated with syndromes (see Fragile X syndrome, Down syndrome, and cerebral palsy)	High refractive errors Strabismus Amblyopia Accommodative deficits Oculomotor dysfunction Visual–perceptual deficits
Down's syndrome[e]	A genetic disorder in which individuals have one extra chromosome (47, instead of the usual 46) with chromosome 21 involved. A broad range of cognitive abilities are found, with some level of mental retardation common. Characteristic physical features include prominent epicanthal folds, oblique eyelid orientations, high cheekbones, anteroposterior	High refractive errors Strabismus Nystagmus Obliquely slanted eyelids Prominent epicanthal folds Cataracts Keratoconus Brushfield spots Perceptual deficits

Category	Description/Cause	Associated Ocular Anomalies
	flattening of the skull, small and low-set ears, protruding tongue, palmar (simian) crease, and hypotonic musculature	
Fragile X syndrome[f]	An X-linked genetic disorder, occurring more commonly in males than females. Moderate to severe mental retardation and autistic-like behaviors (e.g., gaze avoidance, attentional disorders) are common	High refractive errors Strabismus Nystagmus Perceptual deficits
Developmentally disabled[d]	Characterized by disturbances of developmental rates and sequences including delays, arrests, regressions, and atypical responses	Strabismus High refractive errors Visual–perceptual deficits
Learning disabled[g]	Significant difficulty in listening, speaking, reading, writing, reasoning, or mathematical skills. Often, but not always, accompanied by hyperactivity and attentional disorders	Hyperopia Binocular anomalies Oculomotor anomalies Perceptual deficits
Emotionally disabled[h]	Significant emotional problems can result in difficulties in school, work, and social functioning. They often take the form of behavioral problems	Hysterical blindness Tubular visual fields Strabismus Binocular anomalies Amblyopia Oculomotor anomalies Accommodative deficits Reduced dark adaptation Psychogenic visual disturbances Perceptual deficits
Head trauma and injury[i]	Head trauma can occur as a result of strokes, automobile accidents, occupational injuries, and other trauma	Strabismus Binocular deficits Diplopia Accommodative deficits Oculomotor anomalies Nystagmus Visual field deficits Visual–perceptual deficits

[a]For further information, see Ettinger (1991).
[b]For further information, see Alexander (1973).
[c]For further information, see Scharre and Creedon (1992).
[d]For further information, see Edwards et al. (1972).
[e]For further information, see Maino et al. (1990a).
[f]For further information, see Maino et al. (1990b).
[g]For further information, see Solan (1990).
[h]For further information, see Groffman (1984).
[i]For further information, see Falk and Aksionoff (1992).

(Ettinger 1991). Vision and vision-related performance are frequently affected, so optometrists can provide useful services to these patients.

Many health care professionals are intimidated by a patient's special needs. Some patients are nonverbal, and the health care professional needs to be observant to assess how to conduct testing. Another obstacle is understanding the terminology used to describe deficits that result from cerebral palsy. To work with patients and communicate with other health care professionals, an understanding of these terms is essential (Table 17.2).

> Patty is a 10-year-old child with cerebral palsy. She is paraplegic, and uses a wheelchair. She is mildly mentally retarded, and demonstrates good language skills, but she does not read. A report from special educators says that she likes to listen to music and she is cooperative in the classroom. The optometrist is asked to evaluate her ocular skills, and to provide any suggestions that can help the teachers assist her in the classroom.
>
> Since this patient is not able to read, the doctor assesses visual acuities using a Broken Wheel test. The doctor finds that she is a constant right esotrope (30Δ). Her ocular motilities are jerky. There is a limitation in moving both eyes to the left, indicating a left lateral gaze palsy in both eyes. Refractive testing indicates a prescription of –4.50 –0.50 × 175 in the right eye and –4.00 –0.75 × 180 in the left eye. The child's mother indicates that this is Patty's first eye examination, so she has never worn a correction. Dilated fundus examination, biomicroscopy, and tonometry (using a hand-held slit lamp and tonometer) reveal no ocular pathology.
>
> The doctor writes a prescription for Patty for glasses for full-time wear and recommends a program to practice tracking in the classroom and at home, to address the child's oculomotor dysfunction. In a report to the special educators, the doctor reports and explains the presence of the left lateral gaze palsy. Since the child has difficulty moving her eyes all the way to the left, it is recommended that objects be presented either straight ahead, or to Patty's right, but not to her left. The optometrist also explains the esotropia. Since patching therapies for strabismus are not generally considered effective in the cerebral palsy population, vision therapy for this particular problem is not initiated.

Table 17.2 Portion of the body affected in cerebral palsy

Hemiplegia—damage affects one side of the body

Quadriplegia—damage affects all four extremities

Paraplegia—damage affects both legs, with a relative or complete sparing of the arms

Diplegia—damage is characterized by a predominant involvement of both legs, but all four extremities are involved

Monoplegia—damage affects only one limb, either an arm or leg; this classification is very rare

Triplegia—damage affects three limbs; this classification is very rare

By providing a prescription for a refractive correction, addressing the oculomotor dysfunction, and explaining the lateral gaze palsy to the teachers, the doctor has helped the educators understand Patty's visual status. The doctor's report to the educational team includes a full evaluation and explanation of the ocular findings.

MENTAL RETARDATION

Mental retardation occurs at a prevalence of 3% in the United States (Goldman 1992). It can result from genetic abnormalities, trauma, hypoxia, prenatal infection, prematurity, metabolic disease, toxics, and neurological disease.

The extent of impairment varies tremendously. Categories used by the American Psychiatric Association to describe various levels of mental retardation are borderline (I.Q. of 71 to 84), mild (I.Q. of 50 to 70), moderate (I.Q. of 35 to 49), severe (I.Q. of 20 to 34), and profound (I.Q. below 20). Patients in the mild category are usually considered "educable" because they are able to acquire basic skills. Patients in the moderate category of mental retardation, and some in the severe group, are referred to as "trainable" because of their ability to learn various nonsymbolic tasks that do not require reading, writing, or arithmetic. When working with these patients, it is important to consider any associated motor and speech problems that are present. Many of these patients can respond appropriately to clinical testing if given a little extra time to respond, or a little extra care and encouragement.

The most common genetic disorder leading to mental retardation is Down's syndrome. Patterns of ocular signs of Down syndrome have been described (see Table 17.1). By knowing how to interact with the patient, and what ocular signs are commonly found, the eye care professional can have a significant effect in identifying and addressing visual problems in patients with Down syndrome.

Mandy is a 3-year-old child with Down syndrome. She is moderately mentally retarded, and the parents indicate that a hearing problem has recently been identified. The child demonstrates questionable visual awareness, and the parents are not sure how well she sees. This is her first eye examination. The doctor uses brightly colored targets to maintain the child's attention during the examination sequence. Since this patient is not very responsive verbally, the doctor must rely on objective test results.

The doctor finds a prescription of −7.50 −2.50 × 10 in the right eye and −7.00 −2.00 × 15 in the left eye. A cataract is identified in the right eye. The child demonstrates nystagmus and jerky ocular motilities. Except for the findings mentioned, no other signs of pathology are present. The doctor prescribes glasses for constant wear and initiates a consultation with an ophthalmologist for cataract removal. If no other medical contraindications for surgery are present, cataract extraction will be considered.

COMMUNICATING WITH NONVERBAL PATIENTS

One of the greater challenges for health care professionals who are not used to working with patients with special needs is working with patients who are nonverbal. If a patient is nonverbal, that does not mean that the patient cannot communicate. In fact, as long as the patient can blink an eye, or wiggle a toe, communication is possible.

Technology has paved the way for a variety of alternative communication devices. Communication boards used to be the most common communication technique for nonverbal patients (Figure 17.1). These are flat sheet-like surfaces that provide a set of pictures and/or letters. Patients can point to the pictures or letters of their choice. Now there are a variety of touch-activated devices and eye gaze devices that use digitized and synthesized speech. In touch-activated systems, patients point with a finger to a response on a board with a variety of choices; as they point, the word is verbalized out loud by a digitized or synthesized voice controlled within the system. For patients who are not able to use their hands, many of these systems can now be light-activated. Patients wear a headband with a light

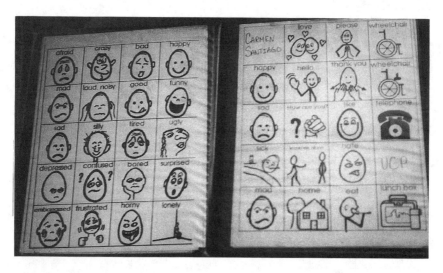

Figure 17.1 Communication boards are used to help nonverbal patients express messages.

source (much like a binocular indirect ophthalmoscope headset), and by moving the head, they aim the light at the appropriate response. To use these systems for communication, the health care professional need only be flexible and open to learning about how patients use these systems.

> Barbara is a 19-year-old who suffered brain injury in an automobile accident. She uses a wheel chair, and her speech has been severely affected. Barbara's communication board has a series of pictures, in addition to the letters of the alphabet. When the doctor asks her if she is having any problems, she points to a picture of a book. "Are you having trouble reading?" the doctor asks, and the patient nods her head affirmatively. When taking visual acuities, Barbara points to the letters on her communication board. When the doctor performs the subjective examination, he asks Barbara to point to the letter "B" for better and "W" for worse. During binocular testing, the doctor asks her to raise her hand when the letters double and lower her hand when they become one again. Ocular testing requires hand-held equipment, but no special responses from the patient. So, the patient has not said a word, but she has communicated and participated in the full examination.

LEARNING DISABILITIES

The National Joint Committee for Learning Disabilities defines learning disabilities as a "generic term" that refers to a heterogeneous group of disorders that result in significant difficulties in listening, speaking, reading, spelling, writing, reasoning, or arithmetic. A key part of this definition is "heterogeneous." Each individual is unique, and has to be assessed individually.

Individuals with learning disabilities may have deficits in visual perceptual, visual–motor, auditory perceptual, fine motor, and gross motor skills. Individuals may demonstrate difficulty with spatial relations. In some, cognitive abilities are affected. Some are characterized as having attention deficit disorders.

For some, the problem may be related to simultaneous processing, and for others it may be related to successive processing. Simultaneous processing involves two characteristic features. Information arrives in the brain spatially, and all parts are available at the same time. An example is asking someone to copy a picture of a geometric shape. The picture is available in its entirety at the same time. Successive processing, sometimes referred to as sequential processing, involves information that arrives in the brain serially and successively. An example is asking someone to remember a series of unrelated words. Stimuli for successive processing are temporal, instead of spatial, and are not present at the same time. Spatial perception is more dependent on simultaneous processing, and verbal skills are more dependent on successive processing of information (Solan 1990).

Patients who have problems with successive processing may have difficulties following directions that contain multiple steps. When the doctor is providing instructions for procedures with multiple steps (e.g., contact lens cleaning and care, use of Amsler grid), these deficits should be considered. Solan points out that individuals with inadequate directionality may have difficulties with phoria measurements, and those with poor auditory skills may require questions to be repeated.

Some individuals may learn and process information better with visual stimuli, some with auditory stimuli, and some with tactual stimuli. (See Chapter 8 for a further discussion of learning styles.) By observing how patients respond to verbal, written, and tactual stimuli, the doctor can assess how to communicate most effectively. The health care professional who works with these patients needs to take these differences into account in developing appropriate management strategies. In addition, strategies for patient education must address the patient's learning styles and strengths.

> Yvonne is a learning-disabled individual who has just received her first pair of contact lenses. The doctor is teaching her about contact lens insertion and removal. In interacting with the patient, the doctor observes that she seems uncertain when presented with written instructions, but she follows verbal instructions easily. As a result, she is given written instructions to use and take home with her, but the doctor spends the majority of the time concentrating on verbal instructions. Tactual information is also provided by giving feedback as she practices. Most importantly, the doctor plans extra time to allow her to practice.

EMOTIONAL DISABILITIES

Like learning disabilities, the area of emotional disabilities encompasses a broad array of problems. The breadth of conditions that can cause emotional disorders is exemplified by the diversity of classifications listed in the *Diagnostic and Statistical Manual of Mental Disorders* (DSM-III-R) (1987) of the American Psychiatric Association (see Chapter 15). Individuals with emotional disabilities manifest a wide range of difficulties and personal challenges. These problems often interfere with school, work, and social functioning.

Children who have been diagnosed as emotionally disturbed are generally placed in special classes with others in the same category. Since each child may present with a different profile, the groups are heterogeneous. A common theme that joins them is a decrease in function resulting from emotional problems. A number of psychological problems (see Chapter 15) may be present. In many cases, by making the child comfortable and allowing adequate time to respond to questions, the doctor can perform a full examination. In cases when behavioral problems occur, the doctor may find it necessary to end the session and have the patient return at a later date to complete the exam.

The optometrist can help these individuals by performing thorough case histories and comprehensive examinations. Ask what kind of class these children are in, what assistance they are getting for their emotional problems, and what other medical problems exist. It is important to know that the emotional problem is the primary diagnosis, and that other unidentified problems are not present. Medical problems and learning disabilities that are unexposed can cause children to manifest behavioral problems that can be confused with emotional problems. A child who has a learning disability, but is in a class for emotionally disturbed children, may not be receiving the help needed for the learning problem.

A wide range of visual problems has been associated with individuals who have emotional problems. These include hysterical blindness, tubular visual fields, strabismus, binocular problems, amblyopia, oculomotor anomalies, accommodative deficits, reduced dark adaptation, and perceptual difficulties. Visual conversion reaction involving reduced visual acuity and tubular visual fields has been discussed. Visual problems such as hysterical blepharospasm, psychogenic color vision deficits, and night blindness have also been reported (Groffman 1984; Schlaegel 1957).

In addition to identifying any refractive, binocular, and ocular health problems, perceptual and developmental testing can help reveal crucial problems that must be addressed.

Many individuals with emotional disturbances display interpersonal problems, sometimes demonstrating reserved, depressed, nervous, or aggressive behavior. They are often fearful of strangers. These qualities can affect the doctor–patient interaction. Provide the patient with a secure environment and a safe feeling. Avoid surprises, and always explain what you are doing. Plan to spend extra time with these patients. When eye contact is poor, therapeutic touch can frequently help the doctor form a bond with the child.

Cindy is a 9-year-old child in a class for emotionally disturbed children. She frequently exhibits behavior problems in the classroom, and the teacher indicates in a referral letter that she does not perform adequately in her assignments. Her mother expresses concern about her development, and has consulted an optometrist for assistance. This is Cindy's first eye examination.

The doctor observes Cindy's interaction with her mother and notices that she takes extra time to respond. During the examination, the doctor makes sure to provide Cindy with adequate time to respond. Special effort is also taken to make her comfortable during the exam. These steps ensure the doctor of the opportunity to obtain optimal clinical information.

The optometrist finds that her refractive error is $-1.00 -1.50 \times 85$ in the right eye and $-2.25 -2.50 \times 95$ in the left eye. She demonstrates a constant left exotropia with reduced accommodative function and oculomotor deficits. Perceptual tests reveal developmental lags.

The optometrist recommends glasses for Cindy, for constant wear. A program of visual and perceptual therapy is also recommended to complement the psychological help she is receiving. A report is written for the special educators, guidance counselors, social workers, and psychologists who work in Cindy's program.

HEAD TRAUMA AND INJURY

Optometrists are becoming increasingly involved in providing care to patients who have experienced head injury as a result of automobile accidents, occupational injuries, strokes, and other traumatic incidents.

Injury to the brain can sometimes affect an individual's ability to communicate and function. For the doctor to understand how to communicate with these individuals, it is important to understand categories of dysfunction that occur (Table 17.3). Understanding these terms can also improve communications with other members of the rehabilitation team.

The location of the injury to the brain affects the type of disability that occurs. A lesion involving the language areas, or their connections, produces aphasia. Aphasia can be expressive or receptive. Expressive aphasia involves good language comprehension, but poor ability to express oneself

Table 17.3 Categories of impairment resulting from brain injury

Aphasia: A language disorder (either in the production, or understanding, of vocabulary or syntax)

    Expressive aphasia: Loss of ability to convey thoughts through speech

    Receptive aphasia: Loss of ability to understand spoken words

    Global aphasia: A complete loss of verbal communications, except for basic stereotyped utterances

Agraphia: Loss of ability to express thoughts in writing

Alexia: Loss of ability to read

Acalculia: Loss of ability to do simple arithmetic

Apraxia: Loss of ability to carry out motor activities, despite intact comprehension and motor function

Agnosia: Loss of ability to recognize stimuli, despite intact comprehension and sensory systems

    Visual agnosia: Loss of ability to recognize objects visually, despite normal visual acuity and function

    Auditory agnosia: Loss of ability to recognize sounds, despite intact hearing

    Tactile agnosia: Loss of ability to recognize objects by touch, despite normal proprioceptive systems

verbally. Receptive aphasia is characterized by impaired comprehension of language, although the individual's ability to articulate thoughts may remain intact. Global aphasia refers to more extensive brain damage in which both speech comprehension and articulation are involved. Patients with apraxia have an impairment in their ability to carry out motor functions, and they may demonstrate difficulty in handling or manipulating objects. Individuals with agnosia exhibit difficulty in recognizing objects.

When these types of impairments occur, the health care professional may need to adapt parts of the examination to the abilities of the patient. Individuals with expressive aphasia are unable to articulate their responses. The doctor can improve their ability to respond to clinical tests by reducing their need to respond verbally. Some patients respond well by pointing to letters or pictures on a communication board. For others, tumbling E charts, Broken Wheel tests, picture charts, and Allen picture cards may work well. When communicating with patients with aphasia, it is helpful to speak more slowly, and to give them additional time to process information and respond. Try to use simple language and simple questions. Closed-ended questions (yes/no questions) may be easiest. Try to eliminate distractions in the environment that can interfere with the patient's concentration. Speak in a normal tone of voice, and do not speak to the patient condescendingly.

When language is a problem for aphasic patients, modifications in testing procedures can enable the doctor to perform subjective procedures. It is important to establish the patient's form of communication early in the examination. This can often be accomplished by observing the patient, or asking accompanying caretakers. Patients who come with communication boards are demonstrating an option. Many doctors who frequently see patients from special populations routinely keep an alphabet board in their office.

Patients with receptive aphasia often have problems understanding instructions, so subjective testing may be more difficult. For these patients, the doctor may have to rely more on objective findings (Falk and Aksionoff 1992).

Individuals who have experienced head trauma often experience visual dysfunctions. These include strabismus, diplopia, vergence deficits, accommodative problems, oculomotor dysfunction, nystagmus, visual field deficits, and visual perceptual–motor dysfunctions (Cohen and Rein 1992; Falk and Aksionoff 1992; Cohen 1992; Vogel 1992a,b). Visual field defects and visual perceptual impairments can interfere with a patient's routine activities and daily tasks. Head tilts and other physical adaptations can occur to reduce the effects of visual disturbances.

It is important for the optometrist to share information about the patient's visual dysfunction with other members of the health care team. Visual–motor and oculomotor impairments may impact on the rehabilitative programs of other health care professionals, such as occupational and physical therapists. Field defects can significantly affect a patient's mobility and function.

The optometric examination of the patient with head trauma should include the case history, visual acuity testing, refraction, oculomotor assessment, binocular evaluation, ocular health testing, visual field evaluation, and visual perceptual testing. Use of objective and subjective procedures has to be determined on an individual basis for each patient.

Case History

It is often difficult to get detailed case histories from patients with head trauma. Patients have often forgotten the events that led to and transpired during their injury. Some have difficulty with speech and are not able to articulate all of the information. Accompanying family members and caretakers can often fill in the events that occurred when the patient arrived at the hospital. They may also be helpful in explaining the course of the patient's condition thereafter. The questions in Table 17.4 are valuable in getting information about patients who have experienced head trauma.

Examination Sequence

Subjective and objective procedures should be selected appropriately for each patient. Some patients have difficulty sitting behind a phoropter, and trial frame refractions are necessary in these cases. Hand-held equipment including slits lamps and tonometers are helpful in obtaining information about a patient's ocular health status.

When it is difficult to gather results, and maintain an individual's responsiveness, it may be helpful to have the patient return to continue testing over several sessions.

Visual Field Evaluations

A computerized visual field analysis is helpful, but not always attainable. In many cases, patients are not able to participate in automated evaluations. Some are not able to sit behind the instruments, and some are not able to respond adequately. When necessary, tangent screens, Goldmann visual field evaluations, confrontations, observations by the doctor, and reports by accompanying caretakers can provide insights into the patient's visual field. The doctor should always try to use the procedure that provides the highest level of information, but when results are not possible with more comprehensive procedures, other less demanding procedures are advisable. When visual field testing is difficult, it is often helpful to give patients breaks

Table 17.4 Case history questions for patients with head trauma[a]

What caused the head trauma (e.g., automobile accident, occupational injury, stroke)?

When did the injury occur?

What type of medical attention did the patient receive immediately, and in the time that has occurred since the injury?

Did the patient lose consciousness? How long?

What types of disabilities or impairments have occurred as a result of the trauma?

What was the duration of the posttraumatic amnesia?[b]

Is there a speech deficit? If so, is it a mechanical or comprehension problem?

Is there a motor problem? If so, has the motor deficit changed or improved?

Is there a memory problem (short- or long-term)?

What visual problems have occurred following the trauma?

Has the patient experienced any attentional, behavioral, or emotional changes since the trauma?[c]

What other medical conditions does the patient have?

What other health care professionals are caring for this patient?

What medications are being used by the patient?[d]

[a]Modified from Falk and Aksionoff (1992).
[b]This has been found to be related to the severity of brain injury, and has been used as a prognostic factor for recovery (Vogel 1992a,b).
[c]This information is used to monitor the patient's psychological response. Patients who have suffered head trauma often have to make major adaptations to physical disabilities and limitations. It is important to identify patients who can benefit from referrals to psychologists or psychiatrists.
[d]Many drugs have ocular side effects, or may affect a patient's behavior or responsiveness.

during the session. When this does not work, the doctor can have the patient return, and continue testing the full field over several visits.

Visual Perceptual Testing

Problems in the visual perceptual–motor status can interfere with an individual's ability to perform many tasks and activities. Figure–ground and spatial relationships, form perception, visual memory, visual sequencing, visual–motor integration, and auditory–visual integration are all involved. A battery to test the visual perceptual skills should be part of the optometric evaluation of the patient with head trauma (Aksionoff and Falk 1992).

Rehabilitation

Successful intervention of the patient with head trauma usually involves rehabilitation teams. These frequently include physicians, occupational therapists, physical therapists, speech pathologists, psychologists, and optometrists. With rehabilitative training and reeducation, many patients can recover some, or all, of the impaired function. The interaction and communication of the members of the team are essential for the optimal care of the patient with head trauma (Chapter 10). Input from the optometrist is a vital part of the team effort.

> Mr. Peterson is a 78-year-old male who experienced a stroke two months ago. He suffers from expressive aphasia. He responds to simple yes/no questions during the case history by pointing to "Y" for "yes" and "N" for "no" on a communication board. He also points to letters for assessment of visual acuities. To answer certain questions, he chooses to write on a pad that the doctor has provided. The doctor notices that it takes him awhile to respond, and gives him extra time to formulate his responses. Through the case history, the doctor learns that this patient is experiencing blurred vision and constant diplopia. Testing also indicates oculomotor dysfunction.
>
> The patient is unable to sit for automated perimetry, but using a tangent screen and giving the patient plenty of time to respond, it is found that he has a right homonymous hemianopia. The optometrist can provide this information to other members of the team who are working with the patient. Making the patient conscious of areas of visual field loss is also helpful as part of the rehabilitation process.
>
> A program of vision therapy is initiated to improve oculomotor function, build binocularity, and improve visual perceptual skills. Visual therapy is coordinated with the patient's other rehabilitative tasks including occupational and speech therapy to generate an efficient, well-organized program. The long-term goal is to help the patient obtain his highest level of independence and function. Progress is slow, but realistic short-term goals help to facilitate the process.

RESIST LABELING

Patients with special needs are often "labeled" by health care providers: the AIDS patient, the diabetic patient, the learning-disabled patient, the low vision patient, the "stroke" patient. It is almost as if the individual is "a complaint with a person attached, rather than a person who happens to have a particular condition" (Shute 1991); it is almost as if the patient *is* the condition. It is more appropriate to refer to these patients as a person who has AIDS, a patient with diabetes, an individual who has low vision or a learning disability.

RESPONDING TO THE PATIENT AS AN INDIVIDUAL

Patients from special populations have a tremendous range of abilities and deficits. To interact optimally with the patient in the clinical environment, doctors have to recognize the individual needs of the patient, and build therapeutic plans that address the individual goals of the patient.

Only by responding to the unique needs, concerns, and goals of the patient can the doctor design a management plan that is suited to meet the individual requirements of each patient.

STRATEGIES FOR WORKING WITH PATIENTS FROM SPECIAL POPULATIONS

1. Understand each patient's unique profile of abilities and deficits. Only by understanding the patient's abilities and limitations can the doctor select appropriate testing strategies and patient management plans.
2. Understand the impact that the disability has had on the patient and the family. The responses of family members to the disability, and to the individual with the disability, have a significant impact on how the family will handle the problem. Consider "family-focused" management plans, rather than individual "child-focused" management plans, to develop plans of intervention that are realistic and applicable to a patient's family and environment.
3. Understand the patient's frustations. Children with learning disabilities do not want to do poorly in school. It must be difficult for patients who have had strokes to learn to live with limited skills that were once automatic functions.
4. Understand the patient's and parent's search for an answer. Parents often want the health professional to "cure" the child of the disability, rather than simply to be fit with a pair of glasses, leaving the disability present.
5. Develop realistic goals. Understand that you cannot cure the child's disability, but you can make a significant impact in the child's ability to function. Unrealistic goals set the doctor, and the patient, up for automatic failure. Realistic expectations create a relationship that is conducive to progress.
6. Treat patients, their families, and caretakers with warmth and respect. Remember that it is important to build a therapeutic relationship with *all* members. It is especially important to build a warm relationship with the disabled individual, and to avoid treating the patient as a "nonperson."
7. Be creative and flexible in orienting your examination and management plans to the individual patient. Classes of special populations are heterogeneous groups of individuals. Looking for one correct method, or one right answer, is not practical. Orienting to the individual is essential.
8. Remember that for patients with disabilities, interdisciplinary communications can be an essential aspect of patient care. Interacting with teachers, pediatricians, physical therapists, occupational therapists, and other health care professionals can improve the effectiveness of overall care.
9. Resist labeling patients with special needs. Remember to treat all patients with respect and sensitivity.

QUESTIONS FOR THOUGHT

1. Describe the difference in the terms impairment, disability, and handicap. How is it possible for an individual to be disabled, but not handicapped?
2. What are "family-focused" plans? How do they differ from "child-focused" programs? Which programs are more realistic for a patient's daily home situation?
3. Discuss five negative attitudes that health care providers sometimes display toward disabled patients and their families.
4. A 15-month-old child is brought in by her parents for an eye examination. She is severely mentally retarded, and she does not respond much to visual stimulation. The parents want to know if there is anything you can do to help their child see better. You can see that the parents are searching for an answer for their child's condition. You identify that the child has a minimal refractive error of –0.50 sphere in both eyes; no ocular pathology is identified. How can you develop realistic goals with this family when you can tell that the parents are searching for a cure for their child's condition? How can you help the parents and child in this situation optimally?
5. A parent calls to make an appointment for a 12-year-old girl who is learning-disabled. The child was left back in fourth grade twice, and is still behind in reading and mathematics. The mother calls in advance to tell the doctor that her daughter frequently gets frustrated at the eye doctor's office. She has trouble reading the letters, often confusing them or reversing letters. What steps can you take to make the examination easier for the patient?
6. A patient calls to make an appointment for his father, who experienced brain injury one month ago as a result of an automobile accident. His glasses were broken, and the patient expresses concern about a new prescription for his father. The patient is experiencing expressive aphasia. The son tells you that his father is very frustrated with his recent condition. How would you plan the case history and examination sequence to provide optimum patient comfort, and to obtain maximum information?

REFERENCES

Aksionoff EB, Falk NS. The differential diagnosis of perceptual deficits in traumatic brain injury patients. Journal of the American Optometric Association 63:554–558, 1992.

Alexander JC. Ocular abnormalities among congenitally deaf children. Canadian Journal of Ophthalmology 8:428–433, 1973.

Ayrault EW. Growing Up Handicapped. New York: The Seabury Press, 1977.

American Psychiatric Association: Diagnostic and Statistical Manual of Mental Disorders (DSM-III-R), 3rd ed. (revised). American Psychiatric Association, 1987.

Bailey DB, Simeonsson RJ, Winton PJ et al. Family-focused intervention: A functional model for planning, intervening, and evaluating individualized family service in intervention. Journal for Division of Early Childhood 102:156–171, 1986.

Cohen AH. Optometric management of binocular dysfunctions secondary to head trauma; case reports. Journal of the American Optometric Association 63:569–575, 1992.

Cohen AH, Rein LD. The effect of head trauma on the visual system: The doctor of optometry as a member of the rehabilitation team. Journal of the American Optometric Association 63:530–536, 1992.

Edwards WC, Price WD, Weisskopf B. Ocular findings in developmentally handicapped children. Journal of Pediatric Ophthalmology 9:163–167, 1972.

Ettinger ER. Optometric evaluation of the patient with cerebral palsy. Journal of Behavioral Optometry 2(5):115–122, 1991.

Falk NS, Aksionoff EB. The primary care optometric evaluation of the traumatic brain injury patient. Journal of the American Optometric Association 63:547–553, 1992.

Goldman HH. Review of General Psychiatry. Norwalk, CT: Appleton & Lange, 1992.

Groffman S. Visual conversion reaction. Journal of Optometric Vision Development 15:6–11, 1984.

Holzhauser GK. Making the Best of It: How to Cope with Being Handicapped. New York: Ballantine Books, 1986.

Linder TW. Transdisciplinary Play-Based Assessment—A Functional Approach to Working with Young Children. Baltimore: Paul H. Brooks, 1990.

Maino DM, Maino JH, Maino SA. Mental retardation syndromes with associated ocular defects. Journal of the American Optometric Association 61:706–716, 1990a.

Maino DM, Schlenge D, Maino JH, Kanden B. Ocular anomalies in fragile-X syndrome. Journal of the American Optometric Association 61(4):316–323, 1990b.

Scharre JE, Creedon MP. Assessment of visual function in autistic children. Optometry & Vision Science 69:433–439, 1992.

Schlaegel TF. Psychosomatic Ophthalmology. Baltimore: Williams & Wilkins, 1957.

Seligman J, Seligman PA. The professional's dilemma: Learning to work with parents. Exceptional Parent 10:511–513, 1980.

Shindell S. Psychological sequelae to diabetic retinopathy. Journal of the American Optometric Association 59(11):870–874, 1988.

Shute R. Psychology in Vision Care. Oxford: Butterworth-Heinemann, 1991.

Solan H. Learning disabilities. In Rosenbloom AA, Morgan MW, eds., Principles and Practice of Pediatric Optometry. Philadelphia: Lippincott, 1990: 486–517.

Vogel MS. An overview of head trauma for the primary care practitioner. Part I: Etiology, diagnosis, and consequences of head trauma. Journal of the American Optometric Association 63:537–541, 1992a.

Vogel MS. An overview of head trauma for the primary care practitioner. Part II: Ocular damage associated with head trauma. Journal of the American Optometric Association 63:542–546, 1992b.

ADDITIONAL READINGS

Aksionoff EB, Falk NS. Optometric therapy for the left brain injured patient. Journal of the American Optometric Association 63:564–568, 1992.

Duckman RH. Vision therapy for the child with cerebral palsy. Journal of the American Optometric Association 58:28–35, 1987.

Gutting A. The role of occupational therapy in rehabilitating stroke patients. Journal of the American Optometric Association 62:595–598, 1992.

Krantz JL. Psychosocial aspects of vision loss associated with head trauma. Journal of the American Optometric Association 63:589–591, 1992.

Ronis M. Optometric care for the handicapped. Optometry & Visual Science 66:12–16, 1989.

Waiss B, Soden R. Head trauma and low vision: Clinical modifications for diagnosis and prescription. Journal of the American Optometric Association 63:559–563, 1992.

Examination Observations

Directions:

This sheet is designed as a review sheet for doctors and students to observe the communications aspects of clinical examinations. The observer should check off Y (Yes) or N (No) as appropriate. In the last section, space is provided for observers to fill in answers. The clinician can sit in on a colleague's examination, or, alternatively, can videotape his or her own examination, and make observations from the tape.

Doctor/Intern Observed	*Patient's Name*	*Date*

	Yes	No	Comments
Checklist of Observations:			

A. Case History

1. The clinician asked all of the pertinent questions during the case history.   ____ ____

2. The questions in the case history flowed smoothly.   ____ ____

3. Proper follow-up questions were asked to obtain sufficient information.   ____ ____

4. The clinician listened to the patient's responses.   ____ ____

5. The patient seemed at ease in talking to the doctor.   ____ ____

Doctor/Intern Observed	*Patient's Name*	*Date*

	Yes	No	Comments

Checklist of Observations: *(continued)*

B. Testing

    1. The clinician gave proper instructions during testing so the patient knew what to do for each test. ____ ____

    2. The clinician addressed any questions the patient had during testing, and provided adequate explanations that the patient could understand. ____ ____

    3. The clinician was sensitive to the patient's comfort during the examination (e.g., setting up instruments at proper height). ____ ____

C. Case Disposition

    1. The clinician explained the diagnosis (diagnoses) in a way that the patient could understand, and that was meaningful to the patient. ____ ____

    2. The clinician explained the management plan in a way that the patient could understand, and that was meaningful to the patient. ____ ____

    3. The clinician provided adequate patient education. ____ ____

D. General Observations

1. What did the examiner do to communicate well with this patient?

2. What could the examiner have done to communicate *better* with this patient? Were there any aspects of the examination that you noticed that could have been handled more effectively?

3. What did the doctor do to *establish* and *build* rapport with this patient?

4. Do you think the patient will follow through with the doctor's recommendations? (If yes, what do you think the doctor did that will strengthen patient compliance? If no, what else could the doctor have done to build patient compliance?)

5. Do you have any other comments on your observations of this examination?

Appendix B

Clinical Interviewing

Appendix B.1

Basic Questions for Primary Care Optometric Interview

Patient Profile
Name
Age
Date of birth
Race/ethnic origin
Occupation
Avocation

Chief Complaint
What brings you in today?
or
How can I help you today? (with appropriate follow-up questions)

Patient's Ocular Status and Visual Demands
Do you see well at distance (e.g., driving, movies, television)?
Do you see well at near (e.g., reading, writing)?
Do you currently wear glasses? (If yes, does patient see well with glasses at appropriate distances?)
Have you ever worn glasses? contact lenses?
Do you experience any headaches?
Do you experience any eyepain?
Do you experience any flashes of light?

Do you experience any floaters?

Do you experience any itching?

Do you experience any redness?

Do you experience any tearing?

Do you experience any burning?

Do you experience any double vision?

What kind of work do you do? (How do you use your eyes at work?)

What kind of hobbies do you have? (How do you use your eyes in leisure activities?)

Patient's Ocular History

When was your last eye examination?

When did you get your current glasses?

or

Have you ever worn glasses?

Have you ever worn contact lenses?

Have you ever had any eye injuries or trauma?

Have you ever worn an eye patch?

Have you ever had vision therapy?

Have you ever had any eye surgery?

Have you ever been told that you have any eye diseases, like glaucoma?

Family Ocular History

Does anyone in your family have any eye diseases, like glaucoma?

Is there any history of significant visual problems, including blindness, in your family?

Patient's General Medical History

When was your last physical examination?

Do you have any medical problems, like diabetes or hypertension?

Are you currently taking any medications (name of medication, dose, patient's understanding of purpose)?

Do you have any allergies?

Family Medical History

Does anyone in your family have any medical problems, like diabetes or hypertension?

Is there anything else that you feel that I should know about your eyes or your health?

Appendix B.2

Follow-up Questions on Symptoms

Severity—Mild, moderate, severe

Onset—Sudden or gradual

Quality—Patient descriptions of symptoms (e.g., dull, sharp, throbbing pain)

Location—Where does it hurt in the eye?

Duration—How long has patient had this problem?

Frequency—Constant vs. intermittent

Change—Any changes in symptoms over time? progress?

Associated factors—Accompanying headache, discharge to eyes, pain?

History—Have you had this problem before? How was it handled? Is there any family history of the problem?

Modifying factors

   —Think: "Better/Worse"; "Remedy/Intensifier"

   —What makes the problem better (aspirin, rest, cool compresses)?

   —What makes the problem worse (rubbing eyes, reading, "midterm" or "finals" week, allergy season)?

Contact Lens Interview

How long have you been wearing lenses?

What type of lenses do you wear (e.g., soft, gas permeable, hard)?

Do you currently have any problems with your lenses?

Do you see well with your lenses at distance?

Do you see well with your lenses at near?

Are your lenses comfortable?

What is your wearing schedule?
  Number of hours per day; extended wear versus daily wear.
  If disposable lenses, how often do you replace lenses?

How do you clean and disinfect your lenses?

How old are your current lenses?

Appropriate follow-up questions to the above should be asked.

Appropriate ocular health and general medical questions from the primary care interview also should be asked, if they have not already been asked at a primary care visit.

Vision Therapy Interview

What type of problem have you been experiencing?

How long have you had this problem?

Describe the symptoms that you experience.

What are you doing when the symptoms occur?

How long do you have to be (working, reading, writing, etc.) for these symptoms to occur?

What do you do when they occur? What makes the symptoms better? What makes them worse?

Have you ever had this problem before? What was done for it?

Who treated you for it? Was it resolved at that time?

Have you ever had vision therapy?

Have you ever worn a patch?

Have you ever been told that you have "amblyopia" or "lazy eye"?

Do you ever experience headaches?

Do you see well at distance?

Do you see well at near?

Do you ever have trouble focusing from distance to near, or near to far?

Do you ever lose your place while reading?

Do ever experience any itching?

Do ever experience any redness?

Do you experience any tearing?

Do you ever experience any burning?

Do you experience any double vision?

What kind of work do you do? (or What grade are you in at school?)

How do you use your eyes at work (or at school)?

What kind of hobbies do you have? (How do you use your eyes in leisure activities?)

If the patient is a child, appropriate questions from the pediatric history also should be asked (e.g., child's best and worst subjects in school, birth history, developmental milestones).

Appropriate ocular history and general medical questions also should be asked.

Appendix B.5

Low Vision Interview

Many of the typical case history questions, listed under the primary care optometric case history, are also appropriate for the low vision patient. Some of them are more effective if they are specially adapted for the low vision examination.

Chief Complaint

What brings you in today? (with appropriate follow-up questions)

Current Visual Status and Function

Are you able to see things far away (e.g., movies, street signs, television, faces)?

Are you able to see things at near (reading, writing, sewing, knitting, crocheting, newspapers, magazines, playing cards, telephone books)?

Are you able to read your mail? price tags in the grocery store?

Low Vision History

Do you know what is causing your decreased vision?

How long has your vision been impaired?

Did the loss occur gradually? suddenly?

How long have you had this problem?

Have you noticed any recent changes in your vision?

Have you ever been treated for your eye problem (e.g., eye drops, medication, surgery)?

Do you have any other eye diseases or problems?

When was your last eye examination?

Have you ever had a low vision examination?

What doctors have examined or treated you for your eyes?

Have you ever used any low vision devices (e.g., hand magnifiers, stand magnifiers, telescopes, spectacle lenses for low vision needs, closed-circuit television systems, nonoptical aids)?

Have you ever used large print books or talking books?

General Health

See Primary Care Optometric Interview.

Patient Medical History

Same as under Primary Care Optometric Interview.

If patient has hypertensive or diabetic retinopathy, or a problem that has resulted from a systemic problem, add: Is your general physician aware of your visual status that has resulted from your medical condition?

Family Medical History

Same as under Primary Care Optometric Interview.

Family Ocular History

Does anyone in your family have the same vision problem?

Does anyone in your family have any eye diseases or ocular problems?

Is there any history of blindness in your family?

Visual Demands

What type of work do you do? Do you have any visual problems in carrying out your activities?

What types of hobbies do you have? Do you have any visual problems in carrying out your activities?

What type of lighting do you use (at work, and at home)?

Are you very sensitive to light? Do you wear sunglasses?

Mobility and Daily Living Activities

Are you able to get around alone outdoors, and at home?

Do you ever have trouble getting around when you visit unfamiliar places?

Do you ever have trouble recognizing people's faces?

Do you live alone or with a spouse, relatives, friends, or caretakers?

Do you have any trouble reading your mail?

Do you ever have trouble handling your finances?

Do you have any trouble shopping for food, or cooking, because of your vision loss?

Are you able to take care of your personal hygiene?

Establishing Goals and Expectations

Are there any activities that you would like to be able to do that you are now not able to do because of your vision?

If we could improve your vision with low vision devices, are there any activities that you would like to improve (e.g., would you like to read more than you currently do)?

Appendix B.6

Pediatric Interview

Chief Complaint

What brings you in today?

or

What brings you in today with your child? (with appropriate follow-up questions)

Patient's Ocular Status and Visual Demands

Does the child seem to have any visual problems?

Does the child complain at all about his or her vision?

Does the child see well at distance?

Does the child have trouble seeing the blackboard, or television?

Does the child see well at near?

Does the child have trouble with reading at all?

Does the child have any unusual visual habits, like holding reading material very close?

Does the child squint his or her eyes?

Does the child rub his or her eyes frequently?

Does the child experience headaches?

Does the child have trouble focusing from distance to near, or from near to far?

Does the child lose his or her place while reading?

Does the child have any eyepain?

Does the child have any flashes of light?

Does the child have any floaters?

Does the child have any redness?

Does the child have any itching?

Does the child have any burning?
Does the child have any tearing?
Does the child ever see double?

Patient's Ocular History
When was the child's last eye examination?
When did she or he get the current glasses?
Has the child ever had any eye injuries or trauma?
Has the child ever worn an eye patch?
Has the child ever had vision therapy?
Has the child ever had eye surgery?
Have you ever been told that the child has a turned eye ("strabismus") or have you ever noticed the child's eyes turn?
Have you ever been told that the child has "amblyopia" or a "lazy eye"?
Does the child have any eye diseases?

School and Developmental History
School:

How is the child doing in school?
Is he or she on grade level in reading? in math?
What is her or his favorite subject in school?
What is his or her worst subject in school?
Does she or he like school?
Does he or she experience any behavior problems in school?
Has your child ever been left back, or had any difficulties in school?
Is your child receiving any extra help in school?
Does he or she know right from left?
Does he or she ever reverse letters or numbers when reading or writing?
How is your child's handwriting?
Do you feel your child is working up to his or her full potential in school?

Developmental History:

Was the pregnancy with your child a full-term pregnancy?
Were there any complications before, during, or immediately after birth (e.g., difficulty with pregnancy or delivery, problem with birth weight, use of forceps)?

At what age did your child first walk? crawl? speak words? speak sentences?

Is the child easily distractible or overly active?

Family Ocular History

Does anyone in the family have any eye diseases, like glaucoma?

Is there any history of significant visual problems, including blindness or crossed eyes, in your family?

Patient's General Medical History

When was your last pediatrician's examination?

Does the child have any medical problems, like diabetes or hypertension?

Is the child currently taking any medications (name of medication, dose, parent's or patient's understanding of purpose)?

Does the child have any allergies?

Family Medical History

Does anyone in the family have any medical problems, like diabetes or hypertension?

Is there anything else that you feel that I should know about your eyes or health?

Appendix B.7

General Medical Interview

Chief Complaint
What brings you in today?

History of Present Illness
How long have you had the current illness?
Have you been treated for it in any way (e.g., medications, surgery)?
Has it gotten better or worse?
    (and other appropriate follow-up questions)

Patient Medical History
Have you had any other illnesses?
Have you ever been hospitalized?
Have you ever been injured or had trauma?
Are you taking any medications?
Do you have any allergies?

Family Medical History
Does anyone in your family have any diseases?
Are your parents living? (If not, cause of death)
Do you have any brothers or sisters?
How is their health?

"Review of Systems"

General

    Have you noticed any weight change recently?

    Do you have any fever?

    Do you feel tired?

Head

    Do you experience any headaches?

    Do you experience any dizziness?

Eyes

    Do you have any blurred vision?

    Do you ever see double?

    Do your eyes get red?

    Are you sensitive to lights?

Ears

    Do you ever have any difficulty hearing?

    Do you ever have pain in your ears, or earaches?

    Do you ever hear ringing in your ears?

Nose

    Does your nose run excessively?

    Do you experience bleeding from the nose?

    Do you have sinus problems?

Mouth

    Do you ever have any problems with your teeth?

    Do your gums bleed?

    Do you have any pain of the tongue or the mouth?

Throat

    Do you experience frequent sore throats?

Respiratory System

    Do you experience frequent coughing?

    Do you ever cough up blood?

    Are you ever short of breath?

Cardiovascular System

>   Do you ever experience chest pain?
>
>   Do you ever experience palpitations?
>
>   Do you ever experience pain or tightness in your chest?

Gastrointestinal System

>   Is your appetite good?
>
>   Have you noticed any changes in your appetite?
>
>   Do you experience heartburn?
>
>   Do you experience nausea?
>
>   Do you experience vomiting?
>
>   Do you have constipation?
>
>   Do you have diarrhea?

Genitourinary

>   Do you experience any burning when you urinate?
>
>   Do you have any hesitancy or urgency when you urinate?
>
>   Do you have to urinate frequently during the day? at night?

Menstrual System

>   Have you had any change in your menstrual cycle?
>
>   Is your flow normal? excessive? How old were you when your periods began?
>
>   Do you bleed between your periods?
>
>   Do you experience any pain with your periods?
>
>   When was your last period?
>
>   Do you use birth control pills or other contraceptives?
>
>   Have you had any pregnancies, abortions, term deliveries?
>
>   Have you noticed any lumps, or tenderness, in your breasts?
>
>   Do you experience any bleeding, or discharge, from the nipples?

Musculoskeletal System

>   Do you experience any pain in your joints?
>
>   Are your joints ever stiff or swollen?

Skin

>   Have you had any problems with your skin?
>
>   Do you ever experience any itching, rashes, or eczema?
>
>   Have you noticed any color changes in areas of your skin?
>
>   Do you bruise easily?

Neurologic System

> Do you ever experience any vertigo or drowsiness?
> Do you ever experience fainting?
> Have you noticed any muscular weakness?
> Have you ever experienced any seizures or strokes?
> Have you noticed any loss of sensation, numbness, or tingling?
> Have you experienced any changes in your memory?
> Have you noticed any changes in your personality?
> Have you ever had any psychiatric problems?

Appendix C

Interview Questions for Potential Office Staff Members

When applicants apply for an employment position, it is helpful to be prepared with a set of potential interview questions. The questions can be divided into five categories: Work Experience, Work Goals, Education/Training, Personal Effectiveness, and Interest in This Position.

1. *Work Experience*

   What is your current job?

   How long have you been working at your current position?

   What are your responsibilities?

   What do you like about your current job?

   What don't you like about your current job?

   Why are you interested in leaving your current job?

   What other jobs have you held?

   How long were you in each position, and what were your responsibilities?

   Have you ever worked in the eye care field?

   What aspects of your job did you perform particularly well?

   What aspects of your job did you perform less effectively?

   What has been your most significant work acomplishment?

2. *Work Goals*

What would you like to be doing five years from now?

What are your long-range work goals?

What types of activities do you like to do?

What types of activities do you not enjoy?

Of the jobs that you have had, which did you like the most? the least? Why?

What do you look for in a job?

How would you describe the perfect job?

What two or three qualities are most important to you in a job?

3. *Education/Training*

Tell me about your education.

What schools did you attend?

What degrees did you receive?

Have you taken any other courses since your formal education, or participated in any training programs?

4. *Personal Effectiveness*

How would you describe yourself?

How do you think your friend, co-worker, or boss would describe you?

What do you think are your strengths?

What do you think are your weaknesses?

Do you like working with other people?

Would you consider yourself a good manager? a good leader?

What type of environment makes you most productive?

What types of office conditions make you less productive?

How do you handle pressure?

How do you handle conflicts with other people?

How would you describe personal success?

What have been your most significant personal accomplishments?

5. *Interest in This Position*

What interests you about this position?

What aspects of this job interest you most?

What aspects of this job interest you least?

How long do you think you would continue to feel challenged in this job?

Do you have any concerns about this position?

What are your salary requirements?

Do you have any questions that you would like to ask about this position?

Is there anything else that you would like me to know about you?

NOTE: Do not ask any personal questions that are irrelevant to job performance such as marital status or number of children.

Index

Abuse, *see* Adult domestic abuse patients; Child abuse patients
Acceptance, of bad news, 69, 70
Accommodative infacility, 103, 257
Acknowledging statements, 32
Acrophobia, 237
Active participation, for patient education, 107
Activities of daily living (ADL), 182
Activity-passivity model of doctor–patient relationship, 81–82
Addiction, defined, 199
Adherence, *see* Compliance
Adult domestic violence patients, 32, 190, 194–196, 218
    strategies for interaction with, 196–198
Affective domain, 18, 21, 106
Affective message units, 22
Agenda
    hidden, of patient, 37
    parallel, of patient and doctor, 172
Age-related macular degeneration, *see* Macular degeneration, age-related
Aging populations, *see* Geriatric patients
Agism, 185
Agnosia, 273
Agoraphobia, 237
AIDS and HIV infection, patients with, 75, 81–82, 187–190, 219
    strategies for interaction with, 190

Aksionoff, E. B., 273, 275
Al-Anon, 199
Alcoholic patients, 32, 197–198, 218
    strategies for interaction with, 198–199
Alcoholics Anonymous, 199
Alessandra, A. J., 152–153
Alessandra, T., 204
Alexander, L. J., 121
Allen cards, 178, 273
Alpert, J. S., 65
Aluise, J. J., 152
Amblyopia, 148, 252, 263
American Optometric Association, 129
American Psychiatric Association, 267, 270
American Sign Language (ASL), 184
Amnestic syndrome, 240
    strategies for interaction with patients with, 240–241
Amsler grid, 101, 109, 180, 270
    learning to use, for home monitoring, 118–119
Anderson, C. A., 1, 19, 46–47, 56, 57, 65, 105, 106
"Angry" patients, 209
    strategies for interaction with, 210–211
Answer-oriented listener, 48
Antisocial patients, 235
    strategies for interaction with, 235
Anxiety disorders and phobic neuroses, 237
    panic disorders, 237

307